ALTERNATIVE TREATMENTS FOR HIV INFECTION

Magnolia Goh, MD
and
Tang Zhaoliang, MD

Science Press New York, Ltd.

Published by Science Press New York, Ltd.
84-04 58th Avenue
Elmhurst, New York 11373

Distributed by TCM Corporation
12490 Central Avenue, Suite 221
Chino, California 91710

ISBN 1-880132-12-5

First Printing: November 1994

Cover design by Bil Donovan
Editing and layout by Frederick Nesetril
Printed in the United States of America

Contents

Acknowledgements

We would like to thank the following people who made up the Edtiorial Panel that advised us and contributed in many other ways

Special thanks to Michael Smith, MD, for his advice and ongoing support and contributions throughout all stages of creating this book.

Bernard Bihari, MD, provided the *Preface.*

Song Xiaoge, MD, contributed the material for the *Introduction.*

Misha Cohen, OMD, Bing Shan Huang, MD, Bo Ping Wu, MD, and Qing Cai Zhang, MD, provided material for the article on *Chinese Herbs.*

Kevin Ergil, MS, Naomi Rabinowitz, OMD, and Michael Smith, MD, contributed to the article on *Acupuncture.*

Mark Proctor, LMT, contributed the material for the article on *Shiatsu and HIV Infection.*

Cynthia Andreozzi, LMT, and Skokie Lee, LMT, presented material and illustrations for the *Massage Protocol To Treat HIV / AIDS.*

Yves Requena, MD, is the contributor of the article, *The Influence of Qi Gong on the Immune System.*

Craig A. Martin, DC, contributed the article on *Chiropractic.*

Nane Cheung, DC, contributed articles on *The Role of Chiropractic* and *The Role of Nutrition.*

Gabriela Bermúdez, MPH, contributed the article on *Homeopathy.*

Dan Kenner, L.Ac., contributed the article on *Phytotherapy: A European Approach to the Treatment of AIDS.*

Fred Bingham provided the material for the article on *Nutrient Therapy: The DAAIR Protocol.*

Finally, Michael D. Anderson contributed his personal experience with alternative treatments in his *Notes from a Long-Term Survivor.*

Preface

Conventional Western drug development has thus far failed to develop effective therapies to treat the underlying pathology of HIV infection and AIDS. Except for some advances in the treatment and prevention of the secondary opportunistic infections associated with HIV/AIDS, the billions of dollars spent in drug development and testing for the most part have been wasted.

The AZT story is an unfortunate example of this. The drug was approved in 1987 as an antiviral therapy for HIV infection in patients with more damaged immune systems. This FDA approval was based on the results of a small, statistically flawed study. Later studies suggested that AZT had some, though minimal, value in treatment of people with HIV infection and more intact immune systems. For these and other reasons, which would probably take another book to reveal, AZT became the standard of care in the United States, Western Europe and those developing countries in which AZT could be afforded. In the meantime, most people taking the drug suffered major side effects like anemia, muscle damage and, in some cases, a more rapid decline in immune function.

Fortunately, a large, long-term study of AZT compared with a placebo was finally carried out in France and England by careful researchers. This study determined that the drug had no beneficial effect on survival. Before the European study, approximately half of the people with HIV infection were refusing to take AZT because of its toxicity, their friends' experiences with the drug and general skepticism about it that had developed within the community of people with HIV. Two AZT cousins, DDI and DDC, were then introduced and approved for general treatment. Neither of these drugs have shown better results than AZT.

The failure of the Western medicine to develop effective therapies has led many people with HIV to seek alternatives. The lack of any effective Western treatments and the search by their patients for alternative treatments has led some Western medical practitioners to observe and investigate some of these treatments. Some of the effective results of these alternative treatments have included: relief of signs and symptoms of HIV/AIDS; stabilization of immune function; control of cofactors and side effects of Western drugs; and prevention of opportunistic infections.

Some Western medical practitioners regularly refer HIV/AIDS patients to nutritionists and practitioners of Traditional Chinese Medicine (TCM), Chiropractic doctors, homeopathic, massage and mind-body practitioners.

In particular, referrals to Traditional Chinese Medicine practitioners have been found to be valuable for some of the following general purposes:

Management of Symptoms: This includes the management of diarrhea, skin rashes and itching, pain, fatigue, night sweats and chronic, low-grade fevers.

Management of Complications: This includes in particular neuropathy and parasitic infections. Some cases of neuropathy have been found to respond to and heal with acupuncture. Some parasites, like cryptosporidium, respond poorly to Western drugs but have been cleared with Chinese herbs such as *Chin Hao* (Artemesia).

Management of Stress: In general, patients who practice *Qi Gong*, *Shiatsu*, and other forms of exercise and massage, tend to handle stress more effectively, as do many patients receiving acupuncture..

Stabilization of Immune Function: The effectiveness of TCM in stabilizing immune function is less clear to Western medicine, because of the differing theoretical basis and assumptions about health and how health is achieved. However, there are a number of herbs (e.g., Astragalus). that have been found to have immune enhancing properties in the test tube. Individual herbs are rarely given alone. Instead, these herbs are given as a part of an individualized, balanced formula to enhance the patient's general health and correct systemic imbalances. Many patients in long-term TCM have reported and blood tests have confirmed their stabilization of immune function while taking these formulas. Controlled clinical trials to evaluate this have not yet been carried out.

Managing Toxicities of Necessary Western Drugs: When patients have seriously impaired immune function (with T4 numbers below 200), Western medical practitioners often must treat these patients aggressively with drugs designed to prevent the major opportunistic infections, which cause serious illness and death in people with AIDS. Sometimes these drugs can have significant toxicities, and these toxicities can frequently be minimized through the use of TCM treatments. In some situations, a combination of Western and Eastern medicines can provide some prophylaxis with little or minimal toxic reactions.

Conventional Western or Alternative?

Recent studies have shown that people in the United States visit alternative practitioners as often as they visit conventional Western practitioners. These studies also reveal that these patients frequently fail to report that they have visited an alternative practitioners because of fear of disapproval.

Only a handful of Western medical physicians in the United States have received adequate training in TCM, Chiropractic and/or homeopathic treatments to practice these modalities. Unfortunately, there are very few of these who have also been able to utilize them specifically over a period of time or with many HIV/AIDS patients.

Many alternative medical systems (TCM, Chiropractic, homeopathic) have demonstrated their validity empirically based on a long track record that demonstrates their effectiveness. Because so much remains to be understood about how to effectively treat HIV infection, it is essential that conventional physicians who treat people with HIV infection become familiar with these systems and work as partners with those patients who are beginning to explore these treatments. Also, it is important that conventional Western physicians work directly with practitioners of alternative medicine, to determine how to integrate these approaches into a sensible and comprehensive treatment plan for patients with HIV/AIDS.

The articles in this book include general and specific information about alternative treatments, their basic theoretical, philosophical and scientific approaches and some of the results of their application to HIV infection and AIDS. This information has been presented for both conventional Western practitioners and people with HIV infection.

Because of the seriousness of the AIDS epidemic and HIV infection, this book is not meant to be utilized as a final source for alternative treatments for HIV infection. This book is meant to be an introduction and overview to the many approaches that are being developed, combined and applied to the treatment of HIV infection. It is not an exhaustive list of treatments. It does, however, provide information on those current, most utilized alternative approaches Organizations and alternative practitioners can provide more detailed information on these treatments. See the Resources section for some of these listings.

Bernard Bihari, MD

Editor's Comments

alternative: *adj* (1540) 1: ALTERNATE 2: offering or expressing a choice [several ~ plans] 3: existing or functioning outside the established cultural, social, or economic system [~ newspaper] [~ lifestyle].

Why this book on alternative treatments for HIV infection? That's easy. I personally know that these treatments work for me. Therefore, I want to be a part of sharing that information with others who are attempting to deal with HIV infection.

I have been HIV-positive since 1979. I am able to confirm that early date because of a blood sample, which was frozen in 1979 by the New York Blood Center and tested in 1984, in Dr. Cladd E. Stevens' HIV follow-up study to the group she had tested and studied for Hepatitis B.

Since 1984, I have remained HIV-positive and, for all of that time, I have not progressed to a diagnosis of AIDS (according to current CDC standards). For over ten years, I have not utilized traditional Western medical treatments. Instead, I utilized: acupuncture, herbs, homeopathics, vitamins, supplements and a diet that ranged from a healthy balance with no milk and few meats to a less-than-healthy, Standard American Diet (SAD). Since 1984, I have had no major opportunistic infections. Because I have not taken anything but alternative treatments, I conclude that the alternative treatments have maintained my health and wellness.

It is almost universally accepted by medical insurance and health providers that people infected with HIV are routinely hospitalized, undergo months or years (if they are lucky?) of expensive therapies and eventually die. Why all of these hospitalizations and deaths after so many expensive therapies have been applied? Is it really the HIV infection that is said to cause AIDS? As the plague marches on, as more and more people are hospitalized and die, it has become increasingly evident that many of the hospitalizations and deaths are occur as a result of toxic Western medical treatments.

Most of the people I have known, who have taken Western medical treatments, have not survived. Their immune systems inevitably gave out from the side-effects of prolonged bombardment of these toxic drugs. Others died from morphine IV "cocktails" given "lovingly" by AIDS care facilities with the consent of families and friends "to relieve their suffering."

Whose suffering? Are these "treatments" for HIV infection and AIDS ever fully noted in medical charts or death certificates as the causes of illness and death? Why are Western medical treatments endorsed and used for HIV infection when there currently is no solid scientific evidence to relate health or survival to them? Why do medical providers, pharmaceutical and insurance companies doggedly insist only on these "accepted" treatments for AIDS? For someone who has been fighting a death-sentence called AIDS for over ten years now, this approach to HIV infection and AIDS is neither intelligible nor acceptable. Administering IV morphine cocktails need not be the final treatment.

When I found a doctor in my health insurance panel who knew about and accepted alternative treatments and non-traditional approaches, he was unable to provide them as reimbursable treatments. Because of a free acupuncture clinic run by one doctor, Dr. Michael Smith, I did not have to pay for weekly acupuncture treatments. When I participated in an extensive alternative AIDS treatment study, which combined homeopathic, acupuncture and nutrients, I was able to obtain non-toxic treatments and free instruction and monitoring for my health. But, for the most part, I have had to pay the full cost of my own alternative treatments, even though my medical health insurance policy is considered to be one of the top ten.

It is difficult for anyone who is not HIV-positive to find a doctor who knows enough about alternative treatments. This is because of the almost universal, insidious bias toward Western medical treatment in this country and a myriad of entrenched economic and societal interests and attitudes. Not only the AMA but most all insurance carriers and pharmaceutical companies and doctors exclusively endorse or prescribe only Western medical treatments for HIV infection. These well-organized and well-financed groups often actively oppose and lobby against alternative treatments at national and local governmental levels. The doctors and researchers who do know about alternative treatments either have learned about them from their patients or have pursued these treatments outside of their Western medical training.

Western medical treatments for HIV infection and AIDS and insurance coverage are biased toward risk-factor tables that have been developed exclusively from Western medical treatments and theories. The treatments and theories do not address the balancing of the mind-body-spirit to promote health. Instead, they emphasize killing microbes within the body, which eventually results in the destruction of the body itself. In immune dysfunction and illnesses, this approach only hastens death. In the AIDS plague, it has resulted in no cure for AIDS, more suffering for people who are already suffering, a loss of time, money and many, many lives. In spite of this and because I have consistently utilized alternative treatments for myself, I remain active, healthy and alive at home and at work. There are little or no side-effects with most of these alternative treatments, except a feeling of well-being, a lessening of infections and a balanced immune system.

This book is not about what has not been done by Western medicine and the AIDS industry during this plague called AIDS. It is about what is being done by individuals and groups of people in the field of alternative treatments at a time when it is desperately needed in this country. It is written and edited for people living with and concerned about HIV infection. It is an introduction to alternative theories and methods that presents another way to look at illness, wellness and HIV infection. It is presented in the hope that when more people learn more about alternative treatments, they will expand their options and possibilities for health and for treating HIV infection.

Be well, be healthy, fight AIDS!

Frederick Nesetril

SECTION I

THEORIES OF HIV INFECTION

Introduction

Acquired Immunodeficiency Syndrome (AIDS) has become the most dreaded plagues of this present age. Because of its rapid spread, its debilitating impact and poor prognosis, people around the world have had to pay more attention to its control and treatment.

Someone in the world is infected with the Human immunodeficiency Virus (HIV) every 15 to 20 seconds. (1) Since the first case of AIDS was reported over ten years ago in 1981, 13 million people have been infected with the Human Immunodeficiency Virus (HIV) and more than 2.5 million people have have died of AIDS worldwide. (2) AIDS has spread to more than 170 countries and regions. If the current rate of infection continues, specialists estimate that by the end of the '90s, the total number of HIV-infected people throughout the world will reach 40 million and the total number with AIDS deaths will increase almost tenfold to between 12 and 18 million.

WHO officer, Dr. Nakajima Hiroshi has said that the speed of the spread of AIDS is faster than anyone could do to prevent it and that there are very few regions in the world in which populations have not been affected. Just ten years ago, no one thought that this epidemic would ever threaten large numbers of people in developed countries. But, the increased rate of HIV infection and AIDS in developed and developing countries has surpassed all past predictions and speculations.

Before 1980, people did not have enough information or experience to describe or even diagnose AIDS. Since medical researchers have identified HIV infection and its relation to the progression of symptoms to AIDS, the incidence of both HIV infection and AIDS has risen rapidly and the number of people who have died has increased dramatically due to the the lack of effective drugs for the prevention and treatment of HIV/AIDS. International and national medical and governmental organizations have already attached great importance to stemming the rapid spread of AIDS. Several western countries have invested enormous amounts of financial, material and people in researching the areas of etiology, epidemic and transmission of HIV. Although there has been great progress in these areas of research, there still remain many difficulties and obstacles in developing effective drugs and vaccines.

Since 1987, AZT, the FDA-approved drug manufactured and marketed by Burroughs-Wellcome, has remained the number one anti-HIV drug throughout the world. Although there are high toxic side-effects and financial costs involved in taking this drug, it still is promoted as the best treatment for maintaining immune function, slowing the progression of HIV infection, and decreasing case fatality rate. A recent *Lancet* article (April 3, 1993) about current research in the efficacy of AZT in Britain, France and other European countries, reported that in a three-year follow-up of 1,749 HIV-positive persons using AZT, there was no significant improvement in time period of progression to AIDS or in survival rate. Since that report, the world press and the AIDS research community have continued to be pessimistic about finding a treatment or cure for HIV infection and AIDS.

The epidemic and plague called AIDS has created much suffering and death for people from all walks of life. One-fifth of all people with AIDS are in their 20s and probably became infected with HIV in their teens. (4) Because of this increased rate of HIV infection among young people, their contributions and resources to our society and our world may never be realized. The World Bank and the World Health Organization have estimated that the AIDS epidemic rises in health care costs to societies and economies will continue to rise dramatically. Currently, the average annual cost for AZT alone is between $6,500 and $13,000. The estimated average lifetime cost of each AIDS patient in the United States is between $60,000 and $70,000. (5) Patients in less affluent countries would never be able to afford many of the medical treatments currently used for AIDS. In many Third-World countries, patients can afford *less than $5 per year for all medical health care costs.* The impact of AIDS in both developing and developed countries can be seen in the increasing inability to deal with the increased rate of infection. This serious public health problem threatens the economic and societal structures of all nations throughout the world. This threat to our health and survival is due to the reality that no effective vaccine or drug has been found for HIV infection and AIDS.

Because "conventional" medicine has not been able to provide effective vaccines or treatments for HIV infection or AIDS, people have been utilizing alternative treatments to prevent and treat AIDS, such as Traditional Chinese Medicine (TCM), acupuncture, homeopathy and Western herbs, Chiropractic, massage therapy, visualization and nutrition. Beginning with the Seventh and subsequent International AIDS Conferences, participants have increasingly reported on the effectiveness of herbal formulas, acupuncture and other treatments. The utilization of alternative treatments has increased as the plague continues to grow with no end in sight. Medical workers, people with HIV infection and people with AIDS who are on the front line of the plague are continuing to pioneer and discover new treatments.

In the following pages of this book, we introduce some alternative treatments that to date have demonstrated some degree of efficacy in the treatment of HIV infection. The list of treatments is not an exhaustive one. We decided not to present some of the more controversial therapies. We also do not claim that these or any alternative therapies not included here are any more or less effective in the treatment of HIV infection. However, we are encouraged by reports from our colleagues that the alternative therapies listed in this book have demonstrated effectiveness alone or in combination with other alternative therapies or Western drugs.

We are presenting this material to promote more discussion, investigation and formal research and application. In the meantime, because of the ineffectiveness and toxicities of many conventional treatments, we are encouraging all medical workers, people with HIV infection and people with AIDS to select more of those methods and suitable combinations of alternative therapies to maintain, balance and strengthen the immune system.

Notes

1) San Francisco Chronicle, July 20, 1992.

2) WHO, January 1993.

3) USA Today, February 27, 1992.

4) New York Daily News, August 28, 1992.

5) US Public Health Service, August 2; 7, 1992.

Theories of HIV Infection

Although some questions have been raised in Western medical research regarding the connection between HIV infection and subsequent development of AIDS, most researchers think that AIDS is caused by the Human Immunodeficiency Virus (HIV). After initial infection, the virus attacks human immune and nervous systems and destroys the immune system function. The result of the destruction of the immune system is the inability of the body to protect against various viruses, bacteria, protozoon and fungus. These opportunistic infections create further complications, symptoms and illnesses such as cancer, which cause death.

HIV

In 1983-1984, the laboratories in the USA and France separated the Human Immunodeficiency Virus (HIV) from the blood of AIDS patients and proved that there is a causative correlation between HIV and AIDS. In 1986,the International Virus Toxicology Committee of the World Health Organization (WHO) formally named HIV as the virus that causes AIDS. HIV currently is classified as two types: HIV-1 and HIV-2. The virus presents a circular diameter of 100-140 μm. Its protein structure and gene function are not fully understood and further research on its structure and function are continuing. HIV has characteristics of polymorphism and more than 100 variant viruses have been separated. This variation is caused by the virus' antigenic drift. Past research indicated that the shell of HIV changes constantly, which makes it very difficult to prepare an effective vaccine. Recent research in the USA and Britain suggests that at least a consistent part of the fixed shell protein coding genes in newly HIV-infected patients remains the same. If further research confirms this, it would then make it easier to prepare a vaccine.

How is HIV infection spread? Past and current research has repeatedly confirmed three main avenues for the spread of HIV. They are: 1) sexual intercourse that allows an exchange of bodily fluids; 2) blood transfusions and the sharing and reusing of needle syringes without sterilization; and 3) placental transmission to the fetus during pregnancy.

After initial infection, the immune system with its lymphocyte and CD_4 cell production is invaded and destroyed and the competency of the immune system gradually declines. Secondary infections and tumors like pneumocystis carinii pneumonia (PCP) and Kaposi's sarcoma (KS) are able to overcome the body's declining immune defenses. The common symptoms of AIDS can include fever, fatigue, cough, diarrhea, poor appetite, weight loss, bleeding, skin lesions, swollen lymph nodes and various ranges of symptoms of psychoneurosis.

HIV selects, attacks and destroys CD_4 T-cells. It

also invades the nervous system and can affect brain, spinal cord and peripheral nerve cells. HIV is sensitive to heat. When HIV-infected blood is exposed to 56° C for 30 minutes, its infection ability is decreased by one hundredth. HIV also is inactivated easily with ether ethanol and acetone. But, HIV has a strong resistance to ionizing radiation and ultraviolet radiation.

Like all viruses, HIV cannot grow and reproduce in a lifeless, artificial medium. It must depend on susceptible, living host cells with active enzyme systems, energy and aliment for its growth and reproduction.

Pathogenesis

The pathogenesis (origin and development) of AIDS is not entirely clear. Present opinion is that HIV infects and destroys CD_4 T-cells in blood and causes secondary immunodeficiency.

The primary function of the body's immune system is to prevent infectious diseases from growing and overcoming the body's normal functions. The key to prevention is found in the lymphocyte cell system in the body, which can detect and destroy invading bacteria and viruses. Three types of lymphocytes cells work together to protect the body from invading microbes. These are the T-cells, B-cells and NK-cells. HIV infects and destroys CD_4 T-cells. When HIV selectively attaches to a cell membrane receptor on the surface of CD_4 T-cells, the virus' membrane mixes with the host cell's membrane and the virus enters the host cell. When proteinase released by the lysosome dissolves the shell of the virus, the RNA of the virus is released within the host cell. Through reverse transcriptase, this RNA forms a new DNA copy, which conforms to the DNA of the host CD_4 T-cell. This DNA then creates more virus RNA and mRNA protein. After the new RNA and mRNA combine, new HIV virus is formed and released into the blood to invade more CD_4 T-cells.

The cycle for HIV is that it utilizes host cells to duplicate and assemble new viruses. After destroying the host cell, new viruses are released into the blood to attack new host cells. This cycle destroys CD_4 T-cells. Lower CD_4 T-cells is the immunodeficiency that creates weakened or delayed reaction to opportunistic infections in the central nervous system, lungs, gastrointestinal tract, skin and other organs of the body. Other pathologic changes commonly occur, such as malignant lymphomas and other cancers like Kaposi's sarcoma. Many of these infections and cancers, because they occur in an already-deficient immune system , are difficult to treat and often result in death.

The mechanism of HIV's selective affinity to CD_4 T-cells is still being researched. Current CD_4 T-cell ranges for healthy individuals is 800-1200/µL. In HIV+ people, CD_4 T-cell ranges below 200/µL is the measuring point for diagnosis of AIDS. When CD_4 T-cell ranges are below 500/µL in an individual who is HIV+,opportunistic infections can occur and some anti-viral drugs are prescribed. Along with CD_4 T-cell ranges and CD_8 T-cell (suppresser T-cell) ranges, ratios of CD_4 / CD_8 T-cells are measured. Healthy CD_4 / CD_8 T-cell ratios are between 1.1-3.5 with an average of 2.0. HIV+ individuals often have CD_4 / CD_8 T-cell ratios below 1.0 or lower. The rapid decline in CD_4 / CD_8 T-cell ratios and the drop in CD_4 T-cell ranges often precedes opportunistic infections in people with HIV infection. Present research indicates the people with higher CD_8 T-cells have a longer survival period.

HIV can infect brain cells because there are CD_8 T-cell receptors found on these cells. HIV infection can result in myelopathy and peripheral nerve diseases. These diseases cause local nerve damage, general encephalopathy, cranial nerve damage and peripheral nerve damage. The most common disease is subacute encephalitis. Its main characteristic is alteration in the brain structure, inflammation and dementia.

HIV infection is divided into four clinical stages:

1) Acute Infection

Symptoms similar to a common cold (fever, swollen lymph nodes, fatigue, sore throat, runny nose, etc.) can occur within three to six weeks after the initial infection. These symptoms usually disappear in a week. At this point, a blood test can indicate exposure to the virus. This HIV-positive reaction is included in diagnostic procedures for HIV infection and AIDS.

Criteria for HIV infection for persons $\geq$ 13 years include:

- repeatedly reactive screening to test for HIV antibody (e.g., enzyme immunoassay) with specific antibody identified by the use of supplemental tests (e.g., Western blot, immunofluorescence assay);
- direct identification of virus in host tissues by virus isolation;
- HIV antigen detection; or
- a positive result on any other highly specific licensed test for HIV.

People at high risk for contracting the virus through blood or bodily fluids are often encouraged to take the test to confirm the earliest possible diagnosis.

2) Asymptomatic

People in this stage of HIV infection are carriers, with the ability to transmit the virus primarily through transmitting infected body fluids to others (e.g., sexual intercourse, sharing of needles and breastfeeding). Except for being HIV-positive, many of the asymptomatic's laboratory tests are within normal ranges and there are no other physical clinical symptoms. The length of this stage, it is thought, can vary according to the initial condition of physical and emotional health, current and prolonged physical or emotional stress, nutrition and life style.

3) AIDS-Related Complex (ARC)

After the asymptomatic period, people begin to have some symptoms and lab tests that reveal a depressed immune system. At least two measurements of CD_4 lymphocytes taken more than 72 hours apart and showing a value of 500 or less CD_4 lymphocyte cells/mm^3 ($<3 \times 10^6/1$) or detectable HIV-antigen in plasma/serum along with one or more of the following clinical symptoms:

- *Oral candidiasis*, not explainable by antibiotic treatment, within the past two years;
- *Oral hairy leukoplakia* within the past two years;
- *Unexplained fever* (.> 38.5° C) continuously or intermittently for 14 days during a 309-day interval within a 120-day period;
- *Chronic diarrhea*, defined as more than 4 liquid stools per day that persists for more than 14 days during the past two years;

- *Recurrent dermatomal zoster* or zoster involving multiple dermatomas during the past two years;
- *unexplained weight loss* in excess of 10 percent of the body weight during a 120- day period.

4) Acquired Immunodeficiency Syndrome (AIDS)

In this stage, people with HIV infection have very deficient immune system functions. The expanded AIDS surveillance case definition for reportable AIDS cases in the United States and Territories, effective January 1, 1993, includes anyone whose CD_4 T-cell ranges below 200/µL. Clinical conditions in this 1993 *Revised AIDS Surveillance Case Definition* include a diagnosis of one of the following:

- Candidiasis of bronchi, trachea or lungs;
- Candidiasis, esophageal;
- Cervical cancer, invasive;
- Coccidioidomycosis, disseminated or extrapulmonary;
- Cryptococcosis, extrapulmonary;
- Cryptosporidiosis, chronic intestinal, for more than one month duration;
- Cytomegalovirus disease, other than liver, spleen or nodes;
- Cytomegalovirus retinitis, with loss of vision;
- Encephalopathy, HIV-related;

- Herpes simplex: chronic ulcer(s), bronchitis, pneumonitis or esophagitis for more than one month duration;

- Histoplasmosis, disseminated or extrapulmonary;

- Isoporiasis, chronic intestinal, for more than one month duration;

- Kaposi's sarcoma;

- Lymphoma, Burkitt's or equivalent term;

- Lymphoma, immunoblastic, or equivalent term;

- Lymphoma, primary in brain;

- Mycobacterium avium complex or M. kansasii, disseminated or extrapulmonary;

- Mycobacterium tuberculosis, any site, pulmonary or extrapulmonary;

- Pneumonia, recurrent;

- Progressive multifocal leukoencephalopathy;

- *Salmonella* septicemia, recurrent;

- Toxoplasmosis of brain;

- Wasting syndrome due to HIV.

Stages 2-4 of HIV infection are not given time periods because not all HIV infection goes through all four stages. Currently, it has been postulated that onset of AIDS can be up to ten years from initial infection. Although some people have remained asymptomatic for up to and over ten years, others have progressed to AIDS immediately after the acute infection stage. No current studies have been able to account for the wide variations of time for these clinical stages.

Alternative Medicine: An Overview

Alternative medicine is the general term for various traditional therapeutics, natural therapeutics and supplementary medicines not found in "conventional" Western medical treatment regimens. These treatment regimens, often called "natural," "complementary" or "holistic," have been developed from a variety of systems that address not only the physical but also mind and spirit aspects of the individual. In these modalities, it is assumed that each individual has an innate healing capacity that can be reinforced and restored to balance through foods, herbs and other botanicals, body work, detoxification, etc., that has been tailored to the individual's specific constitution and condition. Because they are generally excluded from Western medical school teaching and training in Britain and the United States, alternative medical practices often are viewed as irregular or unorthodox in this cultural climate. However, many people can perceive alternative medicine and the wide range of medical theories and practices it encompasses as comfortable or familiar, even miraculous or magical. In reality, the historic record of the uses of alternative treatments in this and other cultures for a wide variety of illnesses has been clearly documented by students, authors and experts in the medical field.

Early last year, a survey published in the *New England Journal of Medicine* showed that millions of Americans were already using alternative medicine. A third of Americans surveyed had used at least one unconventional therapy in the past year. It is estimated that Americans spent almost $14 billion on alternative therapies in 1990. The national health care bill that same year was larger than $700 billion. People are most likely to use alternative medicine for problems that conventional medicine cannot resolve, such as back pains, anxiety, headaches, insomnia and immune system dysfunction. However, because alternative treatments are not usually covered by medical insurance, at least three-quarters of that $14 billion bill for alternative therapies was paid directly out of pocket by Americans. Besides these out-of-pocket costs, it was reported that 72 percent of those patients who use alternative treatments do not tell their conventional medical doctors that they do. (1)

In 1992, the National Institutes of Health in the United States set up an Office of Alternative Medicine. This office was created to examine alternative medical therapies and their advantages in treating incurable illnesses like cancer and AIDS. Like alternative treatments, the idea of creating this office was originally met with some political controversy. The majority of AIDS researchers and people with AIDS are aware of the need for this national office. Even some congressional committees have conducted inquiries and hearings on the uses of alternative medicines in the treatment of some diseases (cancer, AIDS, arthritis and autoimmune illnesses) when current Western medicine has not worked well. These hearings and the creation of the Office of Alternative Medicine are important first steps in the process of legalizing and publicizing practical and effective traditional folk and alternative medicine treatments.

Alternative treatments for HIV+ persons are very diverse and involve many avenues: acupuncture, acupressure, Chinese and Western herbs and herbal formulas, massage, homeopathy, Yoga, vitamin and nutrition therapies, Qi Gong, reflexology, Chiropractic, kinetotherapy, ozone therapy, urine therapy, aroma therapy, hypnotherapy, biofeedback and visualization, energy therapies and psychotherapy practices.

Traditional Chinese medicine (TCM) has been used to treat AIDS conditions since the beginning of the eighties. In the United States, it has been shown that acupuncture can restore immune system functions, alleviate some symptoms, improve survival and quality of life. Acupuncture and herbal formulas are particularly effective when the constitution of HIV+ persons and AIDS patients is still good. In its early stages and when CD_4 counts are above 200, HIV infection can be controlled with alternative treatments and the development of the disease can be arrested in its early stage. Many reports and studies have shown longer survival periods for patients who received acupuncture treatments. Because Western medicine alone cannot demonstrate longer survival rates, multiple alternative treatments are becoming more popular for patients and doctors. Some doctors have combined acupuncture, herbal formulas, massage, alimentation, psychotherapy and support groups. There also is a growing body of evidence that a positive spiritual attitude and the personal confidence and belief in treatment and survival with HIV infection affects the development of the disease.

Many practitioners and medical workers in the United States and other countries have developed various combinations of subjective and objective approaches to combat this disease. When the first Traditional Chinese Medicine clinic in Britain was set up in a hospital in London, TCM practitioners applied herbal formulas and acupuncture to treat various diseases—from common dorsalgia to AIDS. Initially, the British doctors were skeptical. However, soon after they were able to observe the positive results of these treatments, they began to utilize them for their own patients as well as themselves.

In Germany, "green drugs" (plant foods and medicines) are springing up in HIV treatment. Medicinal plants play an important role in the treatment of various kinds of inflammation and tumors found in AIDS. Acupuncture has been placed on the standard treatment list for 9,000 out of 120,000 doctors in France. For several years in China, TCM and herbal formula therapy have been utilized in the treatment of AIDS. HIV+ persons in Belgium and Spain not only receive acupuncture treatments but also are increasingly requesting herbal treatments. Herbal formulas as well as homeopathics are commonly utilized throughout Europe. In Australia, TCM is taught as a master degree course at the Melbourne Imperial University of Science and Engineering. Increasingly, medical reports published in newspapers and medical journals describe acupuncture and herbal therapies in the treatment of HIV infection. In Brazil and Argentina, where medical practitioners are experiencing a rapid increase in the number of AIDS patients, many native South American herbs are being utilized to prevent and treat AIDS. In Africa, which already has a very high rate of AIDS, Chinese medical specialists are carrying out several TCM treatment studies and have presented several research papers about these studies at international AIDS conferences and in medical journals. Researchers in China and Japan also have studied the effects of Chinese herbs in the treatment of AIDS. The results of these studies have generated larger worldwide interest in Chinese herbs.

Present modern medicine cannot cure AIDS, and no Western medications have been developed that can adequately stimulate the immune system in people with HIV infection. Alternative treatments are beginning to show positive results in improving many patients' symptoms and prolonging their lives. These treatments have extended some AIDS patients' lives by five and six years and even longer after diagnosis. Their quality of life has also been improved. But, what are some of the prospective options for alternative treatments and AIDS?

In *Alternative Medicine in Britain*, (Mikesake, Oxford: 1992), the most common diseases that are treated with alternative therapies in Western countries are back problems, anxiety, headaches, chronic pain, cancers and tumors, HIV infection and AIDS. Although many alternative treatments reported were not considered to be primary treatments and in some cases were considered to be illegal, they often were used as primary treatments by the patients themselves.

AIDS Treatment, published by the Centers for Disease Control and Prevention, has reported on TCM and Japanese Han Medicine treatments for AIDS. At the Fourth International AIDS Conference in 1988, papers presented the anti-HIV effects of Xiao Chai Hu Tang (minor Bupleurum combination) and glycyrrhizic acid (licorice). Since those papers, the quantity and quality of papers and reports presented at international AIDS conferences on the uses of TCM and alternative medicine have increased dramatically. At the Eighth International Conference on AIDS, TCM became a special subject for the conference. In 1993, at the Ninth International Conference on AIDS, there were 54 papers presented about TCM. A special academic organization for TCM that is attached to these conferences has been created.

TCM and other alternative treatments already have become a part of the larger alternative treatment movement within the AIDS patient community. Now, the reports of these treatments finally have resulted in considerable interest and research in AIDS research community.

Notes

1) *Consumer Reports,* January 1994.

SECTION II

ALTERNATIVE TREATMENTS

Chinese Herbs

Chinese herbal medicine is a primary component of Traditional Chinese Medicine (TCM), one of the oldest medical systems in the world. It utilizes thousands of Chinese herbs to treat virtually all kinds of illness. TCM has its own distinct forms of diagnosis, treatment, prognosis and treatment modalities. One of the modalities, Chinese herbs, have been used for thousands of years in the Asian world and for hundreds of years in various parts of the Western world. TCM diagnosis of disease was developed over thousands of years with millions of subjects.

The TCM textbooks on diagnosis and treatment often were compilations of thousands of hours of treatment and debate among the head physicians in China. Often, it took months to determine the physiological effects of an individual herb. These effects had to be reproducible in all people with the same syndromes. This approach of reproducing the same effects in all people with the same syndrome is very similar to Western medicine's clinical trials. However, it adheres to strict TCM diagnosis and treatment principles and modalities. Today, TCM is practiced and debated in a similar way. Therefore, it is not a simple matter for an herb to be added to a TCM book of medicines.

Principles of Chinese Medicine

The primary concept of TCM is that the creation of wholeness and harmony will enable the body to heal itself. The various modalities of TCM have different approaches. Some focus on balancing the body's energy while others focus on improving the physical body by adding substances which balance and change the body materially.

Chinese herbs are given according to *Bianzheng Lunzhi*, which is a comprehensive analysis of clinical data collected through four diagnostic techniques. The patient's symptoms and signs are detected, analyzed and summarized in order to identify the etiology, nature and location of the illness. The relation between the body's resistance and the pathological agents also helps to establish a descriptive diagnosis. For example, such a diagnosis could be "Liver *Yang* excessive, Kidney *Yin* deficiency."

Yin and *Yang* Theory

Chinese philosophy and TCM embraces the concept of the dialectical opposition of two polar principles, Y*in* and Y*ang,* which exist in and constitute the universe. In TCM theory, the human body is considered to be a microcosm of the universe. It also is made up of *Yin* and *Yang*. *Yin* and *Yang* are not fixed entities but are opposites in relation to one another. In one situation, something that may have *Yang* qualities could in another situation have more *Yin* aspects. *Yin* and *Yang* as two opposites interdepend and transform each other. When the body is in a condition that is described as a correct balance of *Yin* and *Yang,* it is considered to be on the optimal path to good health as well as to creating a balanced environment. When *Yin* and *Yang* are out of balance, the body experiences illnesses. Chinese herbs are then utilized to correct the imbalance so that the body can be returned to the optimal path of good health.

In TCM theory, *Yin* is designated as the female, right side, internal, and lower parts of the body. *Yin* organs are the *Zang* organs, the organs that store essence and energy. A diagnosis with *Yin* symptoms could include cold feeling and intolerance to cold, lower energy, pale face, a slow, deep or thin pulse.

Yang is designated as male, left side, external and upper parts of the body. *Yang* governs the *Fu* organs, organs that transport or digest substances. A diagnosis with *Yin* symptoms could include fever or feverish feeling and intolerance to heat, hyperactivity, red face, a speedy, superficial or big pulse.

Five Elements

Another important part of TCM is the Five Elements System. This system describes and illustrates the nature of things in the world. The relation between the properties of the Five Elements are used also to describe the movements and interactions of the body. The organs of the body are described through the Five Elements system as: Wood (Liver), Fire (Heart), Metal (Lung), Earth (Spleen) and Water (Kidney).

Every element promotes, increases or generates another element:

Metal ↗ Water ↗ Wood ↗ Fire ↗ Earth ↗ Metal.

Every element can also inhibit or restrict another element:

Metal ↘ Wood ↘ Earth ↘ Water ↘ Fire ↘ Metal

As each organ system within the body is governed by the Five Elements, each system also governs particular body tissue activities and emotional states. For example, the Kidney System manages fluid metabolism, which the West also associates with kidneys. However, beyond this function, in TCM, the Kidney System also is responsible for reproduction, growth and regeneration. The bones, inner ear, marrow, teeth and lumbar area are all associated with the Kidney System. Lack of maturation, frequent urination and low back pain may be associated with the Kidney System. The will and emotional states of fear and panic are also associated with the Kidney System. In TCM, the Kidney System as well as all other organ systems of the body has specific functions that are unique and are governed by the Five Elements, and *Yin* and *Yang* theories of TCM.

Organ Systems, *Qi* and *Xue*

Besides, *Yin, Yang* and the Five Elements, *Qi* and *Xue* are another component to TCM. *Qi* refers to energy and body or organ functions, such as Kidney *Qi*, Central *Qi*, Stomach *Qi*, etc. *Xue* refers to blood, which is not only the fluid flowing the the blood vessels but also the circulation itself.

The immune system in Chinese medicine, includes

the various aspects of the Organ Systems as well as what is called the *Wei Qi* (Defensive Energy). *Wei Qi* defends the body from outside pathogens and is the internal ability of the body to remain strong. According to TCM theory, the ultimate key to health and resisting disease is accomplished through maintaining strong organ systems and what is referred to as *Original Qi*. *Original Qi* is stored in the Kidney System. This original energy is not easy to increase, but it can be depleted easily when *Wei Qi* is used up and not replaced.

TCM theory views pathologic anger in much the same way that Western medicine views biologic pathogens. Therefore, this negative emotion (pathologic anger) is capable of causing illness in the body when *Wei Qi* and/or *Original Qi* have been depleted.

When people in their daily lives cultivate both nutritional and emotional health, they are better able to strengthen their immune systems and remain healthier longer. Those who do not cultivate nutritional or emotional health or who take toxic drugs usually become very ill over a short period of time.

A person must work hard to retain the *Original Qi*. Exercises such as Tai Chi and Qi Gong are highly recommended, as well as proper eating and sleeping habits. If a person consistently lacks sleep and proper nutrition, abuses drugs or alcohol, or has excessive or unsafe sex, they become Kidney deficient. Some persons are constitutionally or genetically Kidney deficient. When weakened, they are more susceptible when exposed to viruses, bacteria or other organisms, which are the main cause of infection and death in HIV-infected individuals. Therefore, this is why TCM practitioners emphasize earlier treatments for HIV infection to maintain a healthy immune system and to prevent the development of disease.

Etiology and Pathogenesis in TCM

TCM theory regards AIDS as *Li Qi* (infectious evil factors), which include the external pathogenic factors of high infection. The invasion of *Li Qi* into the human body results in a damaged *Zhen Qi* (vital energy, the body's natural ability to resist disease) and results in a deficiency of *Qi* (energy) and blood. *Li Qi* is *a* "warm disease." HIV+ persons mostly have deficiency of *Qi*, blood and body fluids due to excessive toxic drugs, irregular sexual behavior or excesses and stresses in life. When the deficiency lasts for a long period of time, evil factors can enter the body from either the superficial part or deep part of the body. This imbalance of *Yin* and *Yang*, either excess (*shi*) or deficient (*xu*), cold to warm, exhausts (*Zhen Qi*) the body's natural ability to resist disease. With the resulting dysfunction of *Qi* and Blood, *Yin* and *Yang*, damage the *Zhang Fu* organs.(the human body's five parenchymatous or essential and distinctive organs, the six hollow viscera or organs, and the unusual internal organs).

Toxic heat invades the lung and causes a dysfunction of the lung in ascending and descending. When accompanied by a cough, this toxic heat can damage the *Lung Ying* and *Lung Qi*. When the stomach and spleen are invaded, the function of transportation and transformation of stomach and spleen is affected. This creates a poor appetite and diarrhea. When the heart is affected, the mind is disturbed. When the Kidney is affected, the Kidney fails to store the essence of life and a deficiency of *Kidney Yin* and *Xu Lao* (asthenia or weakness and debility) occurs. Later, various symptoms of *Zang Fu* organs appear and the condition of the disease worsens, the *Yuan Qi* (or primordial principle) is exhausted, and death occurs.

TCM possesses a large body of knowledge regarding diseases and symptoms similar to AIDS. Based on research combining both TCM and modern medicine, AIDS can be compared to other infectious, epidemic diseases with similar symptoms. AIDS is accompanied by the clinical manifestations of *Yuan Qi* (or primordial principle) exhaustion and *Ying Qi* (or *Nutrient Qi*) insufficiency. Symptoms include progressive emaciation, fatigue, night sweats, poor appetite and diarrhea. It is very similar to a deficient and consumptive disease. In TCM, it is called *Xu Sun* and is classified as *Xu Lao* (deficient and consumptive disease). Usually AIDS is accompanied by lymphadenopathy. This is categorized as *Lei Li* or scrofula (swollen lymph nodes). AIDS conditions worsen when "evil" toxins are hidden internally and and accumulation of phlegm stasis (mucous stagnation) occurs. In prolonged cases, liver and spleen enlargement and malignant tumors can occur. These abdominal masses and malignant nodule conditions are categorized as *Ji Ju* and *Zheng Jia*, and the phlegm or mucous stagnation is categorized as *Shi Rong*. When evil toxins of AIDS invade upwards to the brain, there may be convulsions or dementia, which are similar to the symptoms of *Dian Xian* or epilepsy. Over time, AIDS patients who experience repeated invasion by external evils begin to show exhaustion of the *Zhang Fu* organ functions. Eventually, there is a separation of *Yin* and *Yang* with *Yang* flushing upward.

Chinese Herbs in the United States

Chinese herbal medicine is recognized as a primary care modality in some states and there are some training requirements that are beginning to be developed. Although herbalists are not specially licensed to practice Chinese herbal medicine, acupuncturists who are trained in Chinese herbal medicine also are licensed in many states to prescribe herbal formulas as adjuncts to acupuncture treatments. Because of this and because herbal formulas have potential risks involved when used by people who have not been trained adequately, it is important to select a qualified herbalist with experience in prescribing Chinese herbs.

Chinese Herbs for HIV Infection

Chinese medicine has much to offer persons with HIV and AIDS. Thousands of HIV + persons currently use Chinese herbs in conjunction with Western and other forms of medicine.

TCM is taken to create harmony of the body. People with HIV infection have imbalances in the body that are treated with Chinese herbs according to TCM theory. Chinese herbs that have been used for treating HIV infection are as follows:

1. *Qi* Tonic

Radix Ginseng, (*Ren Shen*), Radix Astragali (*Huang Qi*), Radix Codonopsis Pilosulae (*Dang Shen*), Rhizoma Discoreae (*Shan Yao*), Rhizoma Atractylodis Alba (*Bai Zhu*), Radix Glycyrrhizae (*Gan Cao*), Fructus Jujubae (*Da Zao*).

2. Blood Tonic

Radix Rehmanniae (*Shou Di Huang*), Gelatinum Asini (*E Jiao*), Radix Polygoni Miltiflori (*He Shou Wu*), Radix Angelicae Sinesis (*Dang Gui*), Fructus Lycii (*Gou Qi Zi*), Arillus Longanae (*Long Yan Rou*), Ramulus Taxilli (*Sang Ji Sheng*).

3. Yin Tonic

Fructus Ligustri Lucidi (*Nu Zhen Zi*), Herba Ecliptae (*Han Lian Cao*), Plastrum Testudinis (*Gui Ban*), Radix Opiopogonis (*Mai Men Dong*) Radix Glehniae (*Bei Sha Shen*), Bulbus Lilii (*Bai He*), Herba Dendorobii (*Shi Hu*), Rhizoma Polygonati Odoorati (*Yu Zhu*).

4. Yang Tonic

Semen Cuscutae (*Tu Si Zi*), Radix Dipsaci (*Xu Duan*), Herba Cistanches (*Rou Cong Rong*), Cornu Cervi Parrum (*Lu Rong*), Rhizoma Cibotii (*Gou Ji*), Cortex Eucommiae (*Du Zhong*), Radix Morindae Officinalis (*Ba Ji Tian*), Herba Epimedii (*Yin Yang Huo*).

5. Anti-HIV Herbs

Since HIV infection is considered to be a viral disease, from a Western medical point of view, Chinese antiviral herbs have generated considerable research interest. Reports and lab tests have identified some anti-HIV herbs. They are:

Herba Viola (*Zi Hua Di Ding*), Herba Prunellae Spica (*Xia Ku Cao*), Radix Trichosanthis, (*Tian Hua Fen*), Rhizoma Coptidis (*Huang Lian*), Flos Lonicerae (*Jin Yin Hua*), Herba Andrographilis (*Chuan Xin Lian*), Radix Macrotomiae Sen Lithospermi (*Zi Cao*), Rhizoma Cibotii (*Gou Ji*), Rhizoma Cytromii (*Guan Zhong*), Herba Lespedezae (*Qian Li Guang*), Fructus Arctii (*Niu Bang Zi*), Herba Epimedii (*Yin Yang Huo*).

Chinese Herbal Formulas

Chinese herbs are used systematically and are always prescribed in formulas consisting of many ingredients. With the exception of Glycyrrhizae (which has been prescribed as an individual concentrated herbal preparation), one herb for one single condition is not prescribed. The main purpose of Chinese herbal preparations is to create harmony in the body, not control of symptoms as in Western medical practices. When Chinese herbs are used in a formula, they will be combined to perform part of the function for that particular formula. The formula's ingredients are combined to maximize the effect of each herb while minimizing the side-effects of each herb. Herbal formulas should be chosen according to the individual condition that has been diagnosed and the general or similar condition for which the formula was created.

Several of the following formulas have been used by people with HIV infection. These formulas are not the only ones to use for HIV patients. But, in consultation with a qualified practitioner, the list and ingredients can be used to match the required treatment for specific conditions.

Enhance™ Quan Yin Herbal Formula

Therapeutic Actions

This formula is taken for immune enhancement and immune regulation in conjunction with disorders of chronic viral inflammation and infection. It is useful for persons with chronic viral syndromes such as HIV disease, Chronic Fatigue Immune Dysfunction Syndrome (CFIDS)/Chronic Fatigue Syndrome (CFS) and herpes. It also may be used for treating weight loss, nightsweats, spontaneous sweating, fever, diarrhea, digestive disorders, muscle aches, inability to concentrate, swollen lymph nodes, low sexual energy.

Chinese Therapeutic Effects

This formula tonifies *Qi*, Blood, *Yin*, *Yang* Essence. It also clears heat, cleans toxins, strengthens *Wei Qi*, clears phlegm, strengthens the Spleen, Stomach and Kidney.

Administration/Dosage

One bottle contains a 21-day supply of 420 tablets containing 750 mg. each of the formula. *Internal:* 20 tablets per day, suggested at 5 tablets 4 times per day. *Contraindications:* Discontinue for a few days when there is a high fever. This formula is designed as a balanced formula for immune enhancement and chronic viral syndromes and it may be taken continuously.

Enhance™ is a part of the Quan Yin Healing Arts Center treatment protocol. It should not be substituted for any prescription or experimental drugs. Enhance should be taken under medical supervision. it is available only to licensed health care professionals.

Ingredients

Ganoderma (*Ling Zhi*), Isatis extract (*Ban Lan Gen* and *Da Qing Ye*), Millettia extract (*Ji Xue Teng*), Astragalus (*Huang Qi*), Tremella, (*Bai Mu Er*) Andographis (*Chuan Xin Lian*), Lonicera (*Jin Yin Hua*), Aquilaria (*Chen Xiang*) Epimedium (*Yin Yang Huo*), Oldenlandia (*Bai Hua She She Cao*), Cistanche (*Rou Cong Rong*), Lycium Fruit (*Gou Qi Zi*), Laminaria (*Kun Bu*), Tang-Kuei (*Dan Gui*), Hu-Chang (*Hu Chang*), American Ginseng (*Xi*

Yang Shen), Schizandra (*Wu Wei Zi*), Ligustrum (*Nu Zhen Zi*), Atractylodes (*Bai Zhu*), Rehmannia (*Shu Di Huang*), Salvia (*Dan Shen*), Curcuma (*Yu Jin*), Viola (*Zi Hua Di Ding*), Citrus (*Chen Pi*), Peony (*Bai Shao*), Ho Shou Wu (*He Shou Wu*), Eucommia (*Du Zhong*), Cardamon (*Sha Ren*), Licorice (*Gan Cao*).

Formula Rationale

Enhance™ is comprised solely of Chinese herbs and is the base formula currently used in the Quan Yin Herbal Program for HIV+ persons. It has been designed by Misha Cohen, OMD, L. Ac., based on her experience and the experience at the Quan Yin Clinic treating thousands of HIV+ patients. Enhance is based on *Fu Zhen* therapy, which means "restoring normality." The formula differs from the approaches used to this date in that it is designed to be easier to digest (protecting the Spleen and Stomach) and contains a greater percentage of herbs that are believed to have antibacterial and antiviral activity on the basis of Chinese and American research. Enhance also has a higher percentage of herbs to tonify and vitalize Blood because of the crucial nature of protecting and strengthening the bone marrow in HIV+ persons.

Enhance has Ganoderma (*Ling Zhi*) as the main ingredient, an herb which is a *Qi* tonic and appears to contain one of the most highly active polysaccharides found in mushrooms. Ganoderma has been used in China to treat hepatitis and cancer. Ganoderma and Astragalus (*Huang Qi*) have been shown in Chinese research to be strongly immune enhancing. Other *Qi* tonics are included for their apparent immune enhancing and energy strengthening effects.

A concentrated Isatis extract is used in high doses

for its strongly antiviral activity, particularly in hepatitis, herpes simplex, herpes zoster and viral warts. It has a broad range of safety. Additionally, a high proportion of clear heat, clean toxin herbs are used for the underlying heat inflammation/viral infection present in persons with HIV infection, Cytomegalovirus (CMV) and other chronic viral syndromes.

A concentrated Milletia (*Ji Xue Teng*) extract was chosen for its clinical ability to help increase bone marrow function, thereby assisting in the formation of white blood cells and red blood cells. It is used extensively in China to treat the bone-marrow suppression effects of chemotherapy. Similarly, it appears to be helpful to people with HIV for the side-effects of drug therapy such as AZT anemia. Other Blood tonics and Blood vitalizers in the formula appear to be important in the strengthening of the immunity through stimulating and protecting the bone marrow.

Clinical Notes

Enhance may be taken daily, as it is a balanced formula. It is neither too warm nor too cooling, neither too tonifying nor too dispersing.

Enhance is used in the Quan Yin Herbal Program in San Francisco as the base formula for treating persons with HIV. It has replaced previous formulas that were not easily digested, and it has a greater percentage of blood tonic and vitalizing herbs. The immune-enhancing factor of some of the herbs is believed to strengthen bone marrow. The herbs contain adaptogens, which help when the immune system is suppressed. Enhance may be used with immunosuppressive therapies for cancer.

Chang and Yeung's study from UC Davis and Hong Kong University show strong *in vitro* anti-HIV activity with Viola (*Zi Hua Di Ding*), Lonicera (*Jin Yin Hua*) and Isatis (*Ban Lan Gen* and *Da Qing Ye*), which are clear heat, clean toxin herbs in this formula. A similar anti-HIV activity was also observed with Epimedium (*Yin Yang Huo*), which is a *Yang* tonifying herb.

For more information about and to place an order for Enhance™, contact:

Quan Yin Healing Arts Center
1748 Market Street
San Francisco, CA 94102

Herb Tea #1

The original formula was created by Professor Bing Shan Huang, based on his study of TCM in treating viral infection. This formula was later changed by Magnolia Goh, MD (China), to address the specific conditions found in HIV-infected patients, and to improve its efficiency. It is the first herbal formula to be tested in the laboratory and in a clinical setting. The results of the clinical setting have been reported to several international conferences.

In clinical use with 103 HIV-infected patients, compared with 40 patients on AZT and not herbs, the results showed:

1) Patients taking Herb Tea #1 for six to twelve months had an improvement of 58.02 percent to 87.34 percent with main symptoms such as fatigue, weight loss, diarrhea, and were better than the AZT group ($P>0.01$-0.05).

2) On weight change, the herb group increased to 49.51 percent compared with the AZT group, 37.50 percent ($P>0.05$).

3) No side-effects or toxic reactions were reported with the group of patients taking Herb Tea #1 compared with the side-effects of the AZT group.

Since September of 1991, one non-profit nursing facility for AIDS patients in New York City began to use Herb Tea #1. Up to the end of 1992, 61 patients with AIDS used the formula for different lengths of time. There were three groups in the study:

Group #1: patients who never took Herb Tea #1.
Group #2 patients who took Herb Tea #1 for 3-5 months.
Group #3 patients who took Herb Tea #1 for 6-14 months.

There were 19 AIDS patients in each group. Laboratory test results before the study was conducted were:

Numbers of Patients on Medications

Group	AZT	Bactrim	DDI
#1	14	7	1
#2	12	6	1
#3	12	5	2

T4 Ranges of Patients

Group	T4 Range	T8 Range	T4 Under 200	T4/T8 Ratio Under 0.1
#1	7 to 950	145 to 1,853	9 persons	2 persons
#2	4 to 484	138 to 1,562	13 persons	4 persons
#3	1 to 948	398 to 1979	8 persons	2 persons

Improvement in Lab Tests					
Group	T4	T8	T4/T8 Ratio	WBC	RBC
#1	31%	21%	37%	26%	11%
#2	53%	53%	21%	58%	74%
#3	37%	26%	53%	47%	53%

Weight Change		
Group	Gain 5 lbs. +	Loss 5 lbs. +
#1	6	6
#2	6	7
#3	8	3

LACA Mice Experiment

In an experimental test done with LACA mice, three groups of ten mice each were used as subjects.

- Group #1, the normal control group with no immunodeficiency, was injected with Physiological Saline.

- Group #2, the immunodeficient control group, was injected with Hydrocortisone 0.4 mg. for 6 days to make them immunodeficient. They were not given anything else.

- Group #3, the immunodeficient treatment group, was injected with Hydrocortisone 0.4 mg. for 6 days to make them immunodeficient. They were fed Herb Tea #1 for 6 days beginning with the 4th day of Hydrocortisone injections.

The results of this experiment showed that:

- Herb Tea #1 can raise the weight of the thymus and the number of TH and TS in immunodeficient mice.

- After taking the herb, the number of IL-2 levels increased in the spleen.

- The herbal formula seems to stimulate the quality and quantity of PFC and antibody production from B Cells.

- It also shows that Herb Tea #1 can help stimulate the activity of NK (Natural Killer) cells in mice.

- The total results show the rise in TH and TS helps the production of IL-2, and stimulates LAK cell function.

- The acute and subacute toxicity tests showed no adverse reactions or toxic side-effects.

The LACA mice experiment results were as follows:

Test	Group #1	Group #2	Group #3
Total T Cell	37.67±7.29	22.89±5.11	30.10±5.49
L3T4+(TH)	26.58±7.89	12.00±3.50	18.70±4.83
LyT2+(TS)	16.25±7.44	7.33±1.58	11.60±3.31
Thymus	44.20±11.02	14.20±4.50	28.70±15.41
Spleen Weight	153.40±23.44	82.05±23.39	91.60±29.66
NK Activity	81.71±14.78	30.65±7.74	42.47±7.79
IL-2 (PBL)	49.90±13.45	25.50±6.17	40.10±11.41

Ingredients

The ingredients of Herb Tea #1 are:

Radix Astragali (*Huang Qi*), Fructus Schisandrae (*Wu Wei Zi*), Ganodermatis (*Ling Zi*), Fructus Ligustri Lucidi (*Nu Zhen Zi*), Fructus Jujubae (*Da Zao*), Radix Paeoniae Rubra (*Chi Shao*), Radix Notoginseng (*Chuan San Qi*), Folium Isatidis (*Da Qing Ye*), Radix Angelicae Sinensis (*Dang Gui*), Radix Elentherococci Senticosi (*Ci Wu Jia*), Radix Ophiopogonis (*Mai Men Dong*), Radix Trichosanthis (*Tian Hua Fen*), Herba Prunellae Spica (*Xia Ku Cao*), Radix Polygoni Multiflori (*He Shou Wu*), Radix Glycyrrihizae (*Gan Cao*), Cordyceps (D*ong Chong Xia Cao*).

Administration/Dosage

Internal: 4 capsules, 3 times per day. There are 100 capsules in one bottle.

For more information about Herbal Tea #1, contact:

TCM Supply Corporation
12490 Central Avenue, Suite 221
Chino, CA 91710
Telephone: (800) 333-4069
FAX: (909) 628-4989

Milingwang

Milingwang (MLW) is an old, secret, Chinese family formula. This formula, consisting of 24 herbs, has been utilized for many years as a treatment for immunodeficiency diseases. With the spread of HIV throughout the world, Chinese herbal practitioners began to utilize this formula. Although no large studies of this formula have been undertaken with people who are infected with HIV, a small clinical trial in Denmark, which treated in-hospital AIDS patients with Milingwang, recently demonstrated some positive results.

A lab test done in China in July 1993 found that:

1) MLW enhanced the proliferation of bone marrow cells *in vitro* to mice in the dilution 1:64, 1:128, 1:256.

2) MLW stimulated the proliferation of bone marrow cells after being administered orally.

3) MLW enhanced the phagocytosis of macrophages and increased RBC levels at the same time

4) MLW in 1:100 dilution exhibited strong inhibiting activity to all of the viruses tested in a dose dependent manner. Virus tests included: Adv III, HSV-1, CB3V, Polio V, VSV.

5) MLW in the dilutions of 1:200 and 1:400 inhibited the multiplication of Polio V and VSV.

No toxic reactions were demonstrated in the entire study with different dilution levels.

Administration/Dosage

Oral: 20 capsules per day, suggested dosage is 5 capsules, 4 times per day. A one-day supply is in a small box and a one-month supply is sold in a large box.

Milingwang is now available from:

Milingwang, Inc.
4444 Geary Boulevard, Room 100
San Francisco, CA 94118
Telephone: (415) 668-2933
FAX: (415) 668-3320

RESIST!

Many herbal formulas on the market are ineffective. Herbs which are only ground up and pressed into tablets or capsules have almost no therapeutic effect. The herbs in RESIST! are produced by a hot water extraction method, similar to the traditional decoction (brewing) of medicinal tea, then vacuum dried to a fine, highly concentrated powder and tableted. Each 750 mg. tablet contains the concentrated equivalent of 3,000 mg. of ground herbs, a 4:1 ratio. This method extracts the bioactive constituents from each herb, ensuring maximum potency for optimal effectiveness.

One of the 17 herbs in RESIST!, *Astragalus membranaceous*, is used for depressed immunity in both the East and the West. This important *Fu-Zhen* herb is used frequently in formulas for viral hepatitis, influenza, susceptibility to infectious and cold, ulcerations and sores, and edema. *Astragalus membranaceous* increases the total number of white blood cells (T-lymphocytes), an important line of defense in the body's immune response. The active ingredients in Astragalus include flavonoids, triterpenoids, saponins and polysaccharides. Some of these compounds are thought to play a key role in promoting cellular and humoral immunity.

Several herbs (Astragalus, Ligustrum, Codonopsis, Millettia, Ganoderma and Ginseng) used in RESIST! appear to enhance the total number of white blood cells (leukocytes). Of these herbs, three (Astragalus, Ganoderma and Codonopsis) promote phagocytosis, an immune response in which certain leukocytes attack foreign substances. Some of these herbs (Astragalus, Ligustrum, Ganoderma and Ginseng) may influence specific immunity by helping to increase the number of T-Cells capable of "remembering" foreign substances from previous infections. These cells attack whenever the same foreign substance attempts to reinvade the body.

Other herbs in RESIST! help produce chemical markers called antibodies. B-cells are white blood cells that secrete antibodies. By attaching to foreign substances, antibodies mark invading cells for destruction by phagocytosis. Certain herbs (Astragalus Ganoderma, Ligustrum, Codonopsis, Chinese Yam Root, Peony Root, Eleutherococcus, Millettia, Ginseng, Rehmannia and Schizandra) aid lymphocytes in changing into antibody-secreting B-cells.

Many of the herbs in RESIST! have medicinal properties other than immune-enhancement. Codonopsis (Relative Root) increases the red blood cell count and hemoglobin levels. It also lowers blood pressure and reduces fatigue by having a general stimulatory effect on the body. The major compounds in Codonopsis include saponins and alkaloids.

According to Traditional Chinese Medicine (TCM), Licorice may be useful in treating inflammation, chronic bronchial asthma, diabetes insipidus, allergies, gastrointestinal ulcers, hypertension, jaundice and atherosclerosis. Licorice Root is incorporated into tonics in small proportions. RESIST! contains about 4.5 percent Licorice Root, in keeping with the ratios of herbs used in TCM formulations.

Among the active ingredients in Licorice is Glycyrrhizin. In test tube studies, Glycyrrhizin promoted the production of interferon against hepatitis B. Glycyrrhizin sulfate inhibited HIV reverse transcriptase. This herbal extract was more effective than AZT or DHT in inhibiting cell-to-cell infection caused by HIV-1, HIV-2 and HTLV-I. Glycyrrihizin sulfate also suppressed clumping of HIV infected cells. Compared to other sulfated polysaccharides with anti-HIV activity, this substance gives the liver better protection against hepatitis infection and drug-induced toxicity.

Ingredients

Each concentrated 750 mg. tablet contains the equivalent of crude herbs in the following amounts:

Astragalus (Radix Astragali) 390 mg., Gandoderma Mushroom (Ganoderma Lucidum) 240 mg., Relative Root (Radix Codonopsis Pilosulae) 285 mg., Atractylodes (Rhizoma Atractylodis Alba) 180 mg., Licorice Root, (Radix Glycyrrhizae) 135 mg., Rehmannia (Radix Rehmanniae Glutinosae 180 mg., Sand Root (Radix Glehniae) 180 mg., Schizandra (Fructus Schisandrae) 143 mg., Ginger Root (Rhizoma Zingiberis Recentis) 143 mg., Jujube Fruit (Fructus Zizhphus Sativae) 143 mg., Millettia Root (Radix Miletiae Riticulatae) 180 mg., Dodder Seeds (Semen

Cuscutae) 180 mg., Chinese Yam Root (Radix Dioscoreae) 180 mg., Balloon Flower Root (Radix Platycodi Grandiflori) 143 mg., Privet Fruit (Fructus Ligustri Lucidi) 180 mg., Peony Fruit (Radix Paeoniae Albae) 90 mg., Tangerine Peel (Pc. Citri Reticulatae) 90 mg.

The information presented here is based on TCM theory and preliminary scientific research. These finding should not be construed in any way as medical claims for RESIST! or its ingredients. Individuals with clinically diagnosed immune disorders should consult a qualified health care practitioner before taking RESIST! or any other adjunctive nutritional food supplements.

Chinese Herbal Medicine for HIV An African Treatment Protocol

From April 1989 to April 1991, Professor Wei Bo Lu, Bo Ping Wu and a Chinese medical team gave Chinese herbal treatments to HIV-infected African patients. These treatments were administered by the team to over 400 patients in Tanzania. The following analysis is based on 158 patients from the Muhimbili Medical Center, Dar-es-Salaam, Tanzania. This analysis is taken from a final report that will be presented to international AIDS conferences. All herbal formulas mentioned in this study currently are not available in the U.S.A.

Profiles for the patients were:

1) Elisa and Western Blot HIV + with immune deficiency (T_4/T_8 ratio < 1.0 with T_4 cell counts < 400/mm^3;

2) resident or frequent visitor of Dar-es-Salaam;

4) seven years or older;

5) currently not pregnant;and

6) volunteer for Chinese herbal treatments.

These patients were given blood laboratory tests (Elisa, Western Blot; T_4/T_8 counts and ratios, and old Tuberculosis tests), physical examinations and filled out questionnaires before treatment began. They were given the Chinese herbal medicine for more than three months (one course of treatment). The average treatment time for the group was 320.5 days (between 90 and 866 days). Patients were divided into four treatment categories: (Lung style, Spleen style, Kidney style and Heart style.) Herbal medicines were given according to the constitutional diagnosis. Thirty-six cases (22.78 percent) with opportunistic infections were given Western medications as well.

Herbal Medicines Used in Study

801 muscle injection, 3 times a week; 10 times in a course, stop for five days, then begin second course.

802 drink, 1 ampule, 2 to 3 times per day.

803 pills, 1 to 2 pills, 3 times per day.

806 muscle injection, 3 times a week, 10 times in a course, stop for five days then begin second course.

809 capsules, 1 to 2 capsules, 3 times per day.

810 drink, 3 ampules, 3 times a day.

901 pill, 3 to 5 pills, 3 times per day.

Shen Mai Yin, 1 dose, per day.

Niu Jiu Zi Tang, one dose per day.

Karnovsky Scores

The measurements for general health included Karnovsky Score ratings as follows:

100	Normal
90	Normal activity, slight symptoms.
80	Some fatigue, some symptoms.
70	Self help but cannot handle daily activities.
60	Needs help most of the time.
50	Complete care needed.
40	Disabled.
30	Severely disabled, in-hospital care needed.
20	Critical condition, constant treatment maintained.
10	Close to death, quick and severe development of disease.
0	Death.

Clinical Information

Before the study, the following clinical information for 158 patients was:

- 81 were male, 77 were female.
- 124 (78.48 percent) were between 21 and 40 years.
- 142 (89.07 percent) were diagnosed with ARC or AIDS, 16 (10.13 percent) were asymptomatic HIV positive.

- 101 (63.92 percent) were HIV positive less than 6 months, 11 (6.96 percent) were HIV positive more than 2 years.

- Complaints included fever, fatigue, weight loss, diarrhea, coughs, rashes, swollen glands.

- 19 cases of weight loss were > 10 kg.(22 lbs.) and one > 20 kg.(43 lbs.).

- 17 cases of shingles and 10 cases of thrush were reported.

- Karnovsky Scores of 70-95 averaged 81.55 ± 5.67.

- T_4 cell counts before treatment averaged 186.75 ± 170.94/mm^3. Forty-nine cases (31.01 percent) with T4 cell counts < 100/mm^3, T_4/T_8 ratios < 0.40 ± 0.33, with 26 (16.46 percent) T_4/T_8 ratios < 1.0.

- 74 cases (46.84 percent) of old tuberculosis positive and 84 cases (53.16 percent) negative cases were found.

- X-rays revealed 15 cases of bronchial infection, 3 cases of pulmonary tuberculosis, 1 case with cavity in lung.

- TCM classifications included 78 cases of Lung style, 59 cases of Spleen style, 4 cases of Heart style and 17 cases of Lung and Spleen style.

- TCM tongue diagnosis classifications included 32 cases of red, 25 cases of purple with spots, 76 cases with thin and white coating, and various others with thin and yellow, white and greasy, yellow and greasy, and peeling in the middle.

- TCM pulse diagnosis classifications included 119 cases with a thin pulse, 55 cases with thin and wiry pulse, 32 cases with thin and deep pulse, 29 with thin and speedy pulse, 3 with only thin, 24 with slow pulse and 14 with slippery pulse.

Results of Treatment

1) Antibody positive tests showed some reversals to negative and/or minimally positive.

2) Immune system improvement included T_4/T_8 ratio > 0.2.and/or T_4 cell count increases of $40/mm^3$.

3) Improvement of symptoms: weight gain > 2 kg and some symptom changes from + to - or ± to -, or 2 degrees lower (e.g., +++ to + or ++ to ± or _).

Changes in 1, 2 and 3 were considered "Excellent results." Changes in 1 and/or 2 plus 3 were considered "Good Results." "Partial Effects" included no change or slight decrease in symptoms, improved lab tests with increased symptoms. "No Change" included no improvement in lab tests and symptoms and/or death.

According to the above **general standards of measuring results**, there were 3 cases (1.90 percent) that were Excellent Results, 36 cases (22.78 percent) Good Results, 24 cases (15.19 percent) Partial Effect, with a total effective of 63 (38.87 percent). There were 95 cases (60.13 percent that had No Change with 13 cases (8.28 percent) of death.

After treatment, **Elisa and Western Blot lab tests**

revealed that 7 cases tested negative on the Elisa test. Of those 7, 5 cases were confirmed as negative on the Western Blot test and remained negative for up to one year. Of 4 cases that had occasional positive Elisa tests, 2 were confirmed to be negative with the Western Blot and 1 reversed to negative after 2 months. Only one case reverted back to positive.

T-cell results for immune function after treatment were considered to be positive when neither of following levels decreased and either the T_4/T_8 ratio change was > 0.2.or T_4 cell count increased $40/mm^3$. With those standards, 49 cases (31.01 percent) improved, 55 cases (34.81 percent) remained the same and 54 cases (34.18).

With **Karnovsky Scores**, 13 cases were 0 (died) and 145 cases averaged 85.21 ± 7.61. Eighty-two cases (51.90 percent) had an average increase of 8.11 ± 3.65; 36 cases (22.79 percent) had an average decrease of 5.97 ± 3.55, and 27 cases (17.09) remained the same.

Eight main symptom changes were:

1) Weight: 52 cases (32.91 percent) increased > 2 kg., 50 cases decreased < 2 kg., 56 cases remained the same weight.

2) Fatigue: 50.02 percent (52 cases) improved.

3) Fever: 35 cases (47.29 percent) improved.

4) Cough: 25 cases (30.12 percent) reported improved.

5) Diarrhea: 30 cases (62.50 percent) improved.

6) Poor appetite: 30 cases (54.55 percent) improved.

7) Rashes: 30 cases (31.91 percent) improved.

8) Swollen glands: 54 cases (65.06 percent) improved. Of all patients with swollen glands that improved, most of the swollen glands disappeared after treatment.

Acupuncture

Acupuncture is a component of one of the oldest medical systems in the world. This system, Traditional Chinese Medicine (TCM), originated in China more than 2,500 years ago. Acupuncture, however, is much older.

During and even before the Stone Age, from 4,000 to 10,000 years ago, people in China discovered that a *bian* (a sharp stone flake used to kill animals) could also be more finely hewn into sharp, needle-like stone instruments that could be applied to the body to relieve pain or illnesses. There is no direct evidence of the discovery and development of Stone Age acupuncture. However, it is assumed that acupuncture was discovered during that time, when the sharp side of a *bian* accidentally punctured a part of the body of a hunter. The accidental puncture was found to relieve either pain or symptoms. From this incident came the connection and development of all acupuncture theory and practice that has been handed down over the centuries to successive generations in China. As acupuncture was practiced and perfected over time, the original stone needles were replaced by bamboo needles, which were later replaced by iron, gold and silver needles. Stainless steel needles are widely used today by all acupuncturists.

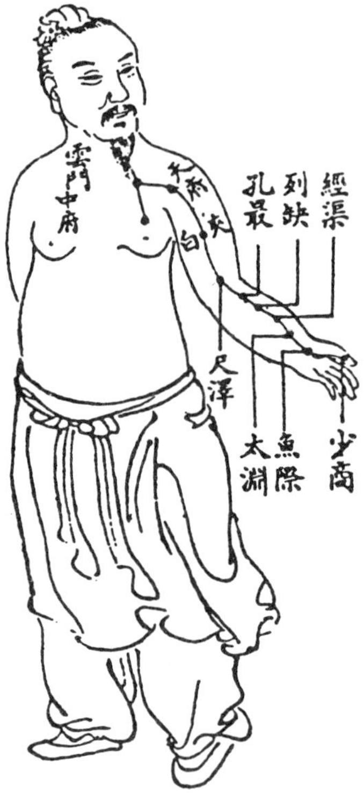

Acupuncture is known throughout the world and is utilized in the treatment of a wide range of diseases. Acupuncture practices, which began in China, traveled to Japan around 562 A.D. By the end of the seventeenth century, it had traveled to Europe. In recent decades and especially the past ten years, acupuncture has begun to be known and used more widely throughout the world as a generally accepted form of treatment. The clinical use and study of acupuncture for immune diseases such as cancer or AIDS has begun to challenge Western medical theories and practices for these diseases. Hundreds of reports are coming from thousands of researchers and scientists in many countries about promising clinical and laboratory results of acupuncture treatment. These reports are presented yearly at conferences and seminars sponsored by the World Federal Acupuncture Society set up in 1987. The World Health Organization (WHO) has set up four international acupuncture study centers in China to train medical workers to use acupuncture for the treatment of diseases. Acupuncture is practiced in over 100 countries today. It is a nationally-licensed form of medicine in all Asian countries and in many European countries.

Acupuncture in the United States

Acupuncture has existed in the United States as long as Chinese people have lived here. Initially, during the 1800s, as immigrants arrived and settled in Chinatown communities in major cities, so did acupuncture. With President Nixon's visit to China, there was an opening up of relations between Communist China and the United States. With the accompanying cultural and economic exchanges beginning in the early 1970s, there has been an increased interest in acupuncture.

In the United States, acupuncture is licensed by 27 states and the District of Columbia. Another four states allow acupuncturists to practice under Western medical supervision. The first states to license acupuncturists in the United States were Nevada, followed by New Mexico, California and Florida. Today, 23 states and the District of Columbia license or register acupuncturists. They are: Alaska, California, Colorado, the District of Columbia, Florida, Hawaii, Iowa, Maine, Maryland*, Massachusetts*, Montana, Nevada, New Jersey, New Mexico, New York, North Carolina, Oregon, Pennsylvania*, Rhode Island, Texas, Utah*, Washington, Wisconsin, Vermont. (States with * require Western medical supervision.) In other states, acupuncture may be unregulated altogether or prohibited by law.

There are many schools of acupuncture and TCM in the United States. Every year, there are many national or international conferences and seminars held throughout the United States to provide acupuncture practitioners opportunities for scholarly exchanges, academic and practical experiences and knowledge.

In theory, acupuncture is used to treat any disease. Acupuncture uses the body's own energy to heal itself. Therefore, the uses and results of acupuncture are often wide and varied. Acupuncture theory is derived from ancient Chinese philosophy, which describes the human body in terms of energy, rather than matter. The ancient Chinese believed that basic life energies (*Qi* and *Xue*) are present in every living creature. According to TCM, *Qi* and *Xue* reside in particular areas of the human body as well as elements of the earth and in food. These energies circulate along specific pathways or channels in the body called meridians. Meridians connect the body's external surface and internal organs as a whole. If the body's external surface or internal organs experience illness, disease or other problems, these problems would affect the connecting channels. By stimulating appropriate acupoints along the affected channels, the *Qi* and *Xue* begin to flow more smoothly in these channels and throughout the organs and body. With the restoration and regulation of *Qi* and *Xue,* pain is released and health is restored.

Acupuncture is the TCM application and manipulation of fine sterile metal needles and/or of heat and herbs (Moxabustion) to specific points (Acupoints) along channels of energy in the body called meridians. The control and regulation of *Qi* and *Xue* in the body along these meridians is relatively painless and often is accompanied by a sensation or heaviness, warmth or movement of energy at the acupoint that has been stimulated by needles or heat and herbs.

Although there is no known Western medical corollary for acupuncture, and although the specific

Western medical, theoretical and actual mechanisms of acupuncture are still unknown, scientific research has proved acupuncture does regulate the function of cardiovascular, digestion, urinary and neuroimmune systems. There also is proof of increased body resistance to infections through enhancing the immune system and the antiphogistic, analgesic, antispastic, antishock and antiparalytic effects of acupuncture.

In practice, acupuncture is more effective in some diseases than in others. Scientific studies have resulted in the WHO developing a list of diseases or symptoms that respond well to acupuncture treatment. They are:

Upper Respiratory Tract: acute sinusitis, acute rhinitis, common cold, acute tonsillitis.

Respiratory System: acute bronchitis, Bronchial asthma (most effective in children and in patients without complicating diseases).

Disorders of the Eye: acute conjunctivitis, central retinitis, myopia (in children), cataract (without complications).

Disorders of the Mouth: Toothaches, post extraction pain, gingivitis, acute and chronic pharyngitis.

Gastro-Intestinal Disorders: spasms of esophagus and cardia, hiccough, gastroptosis, acute and chronic gastritis, gastric hyperacidity, chronic duodenal ulcer (pain relief), acute duodenal ulcer (without complication), acute and chronic colitis, acute bacillary dysentery, constipation, diarrhea, paralytic ileus.

Neurological and Musculo-Skeletal Disorders: headache and migraine, trigeminal neuralgia, facial palsy, (early stages, within 3-6 months), paresis following stroke, peripheral neuropathies, sequelae to poliomyelitis (early stages, within 6 months), Meniere's Disease, neurogenic bladder dysfunction, nocturnal enuresis, intercostal neuralgia, cervicobrachial syndrome, "frozen shoulder" and "tennis elbow," sciatica, low back pain, osteoarthritis.

Acupuncture and the Immune System

The immune system is one of the systems that is strongly influenced by acupuncture stimulation. A considerable amount of research already has been completed on the effects of acupuncture on immune problems (e.g., infections, cancer, inflammations and immuno-deficiency). Acupuncture influences specific and non-specific cellular and humoral immunities. It activates cell proliferation, including blood cells, reticuloendothetial cells, and traumatized cells. It activates leucocytosic, microbicidal activities and stimulates production of antibodies, globulin, complement and interferon. It also has been shown that stimulation of certain points (*Hegu*-L4, *Neiguan*-P6, *Zusanli*-S36) increase globulin concentration. Daily acupuncture stimulation of 7-10 days significantly increased IgG levels in both serum and gingival sulous fluid.

In a laboratory study that used moxa stick to treat immuno-deficient animals, there were increases in abdominal macrophage and phagocytosis (1,2). A study with cancer patients showed increases in phagocytosis of neutrophil granulocytes when acupuncture treatments were given in S36 (*Zusanli*), P6 (*Neiguang*), and Sp6 (*Sanyinjian*). (3) Using acupuncture points of S36 (*Zusanli*), CV3 (*Guanyan*),

CV6 (*Qi Hai*), and B43 (*Gao Fang*) in healthy people could stimulate the activity of NK (Natural Killer cells) far more than a control group that did not receive acupuncture point stimulation (4). Other studies also have shown that the use of acupuncture increases and stimulates LTT, RFC, CD4 and B cells (5, 6). One report on 21 patients with severe diarrhea from bacillary dysentery (bacterial infection of the intestine) indicated the increase of LTT and RFC levels ($P < 0.05$) after acupuncture stimulation once a day for three days on S37 (*Shanjuxu*) and Sp7 (*Lou Gu*).

Interferon is an important factor in the function of antiviral, antimitotic and adjunct immune functions. Research shows that acupuncture and moxabustion can stimulate viral infected mice to produce interferon to help fight the virus.(7)

Acupuncture Regulating Immune Function

Years ago, scientists confirmed that the regulatory function of acupuncture to the immune system occurred through its neuro-humoral regulation. Further studies discovered opium receptors in immunocytes and the production of opium peptides (OLP) and other humoral functions from the immune systems. This led to the discovery that neuroendocrine functions are effected through the regulatory function of acupuncture.

Acupuncture was found to stimulate the release of OLP. One study with guinea pigs found that acupuncture activated MEK receptors and regulated cellular immunity (8)

Acupuncture and the Treatment of HIV Infection

People with HIV infection often select acupuncture initially as their first choice. Even if they do not understand it very well, they may have heard about and begin to utilize acupuncture to reduce pain.

As early as 1982, people with HIV infection, ARC and AIDS have received acupuncture at Lincoln Hospital's Acupuncture Clinic in New York City. More than 200 people were receiving these treatments as well as Chinese herbs for several years. In 1987, reports from these patients indicated a reduction in fatigue, abnormal sweating, diarrhea in a short period of time, often as quickly as after the first 4-5 treatments. Patients usually described and improved sense of well-being rather than merely an absence of symptoms. Some patients have had from 15 to 25 pound weight gains and are able to return to long hours of work. Those taking chemotherapy often reported a decrease in side-effects such as fatigue, nausea, and weakness. (9) The most dramatic and reproducible benefit of acupuncture treatment is that the patient feels calmer and more centered and is better able to cope. (10)

Pain is one of the main symptoms of HIV infected people and people with AIDS. This pain can originate in all parts of the body: general body aches, joint pain, peripheral neuropathy, stomachache, headache, cramps in the digestive system organs and pain from Kaposi's sarcoma lesions on the skin or in internal organs. An especially predominant kind of pain is sensory peripheral neuropathy, which affects up to 30 percent of patients with AIDS. (11) Some medications used in the treatment of HIV infected patients (e.g.,

DDI, D4T, AZT) cause peripheral neuropathy. Peripheral neuropathy is not life-threatening, but it can range anywhere from annoying to incapacitating. At this point, no medication has been proven effective in relieving neuropathy or its related symptoms. But, acupuncture treatment has shown some positive results.

In one study of 31 patients with peripheral neuropathy, acupuncture alleviated pain or tingling in 12 (38.7 percent) of the patients. Another 11 patients from this study noted relief of most symptoms with the exception of one or two, who were only partially relieved. Five others had a reduction in pain with occasional recurrences. Three patients who received only one treatment did not respond. In this study, patients received one to three treatments per week and began to see the result of these treatments within three to five treatments. (12)

Acupuncture Points for Treating HIV Infection

The clinical presentation of HIV infection can vary widely. Acupuncturists must study each patient's history and symptoms, check pulse and tongue carefully, and tailor treatment to fit the individual. Acupuncture really is an art of health. Selecting acupoints is like composing a painting. Trained acupuncturists know how to select acupoints according to the individual patient's condition. It is important to select the acupoints according to specific ranges of symptoms and close examination of the patient's condition. In this short article, we are listing only general points according to the principles of TCM. According to these principles, HIV-infected patients can be grouped generally into six categories:

1. Asymptomatic

This group of HIV+ people have no physical or laboratory test abnormalities. Acupuncture can be used to maintain immune function and prevent infections for asymptomatic, HIV-infected people. Treatment could be once a week or once a month.

Acupoints:
Hegu (L4), *Neiguan* (P6), *Zusanli* (S36), *Yamen* (GV15), *Dazhui* (GV14), *Quchi* (L11), *Shangjuxu* (S37) have been tested in laboratories and proved to raise immune system function.

Auricular Points:
Kidney, Spleen, Endocrine, Adrenal Gland.

Moxabustion:
Dazhui (GV14), *Zusanli* (S36).

2. Qi and Yin Deficiency of Lung

This group of patients have more problems with their respiratory system and skin. Main symptoms include: frequent cold, sinusitis, pharyego-laryngitis, tonsillitis or rhinitis, cough with or without phlegm, shortness of breath. Some people with a history of these problems can go on to develop PCP, bacterial pneumonia or bronchitis. Dry skin, itching and different kinds of dermatitis are often found in this group. Emotionally, these people often are easily upset or depressed. Treatment should be once or twice a week.

Tongue:
Pale or gray, wet, smooth; white, thick coating.

Acupoints:
Zhongfu (L1), *Lieque* (L7), *Taiyuen* (L9), *Feishu* (B13), *Quchi* (L11), *Hegu* (L4), *Shanzhong* (CV17). With sinusitis, add *Yinxiang* (L20), *Yingtang* (EX3).

Auricular Points:
Lung, Endocrine, Large Intestine.

Moxabustion:
Daizhui (GV14), *Shenzhu* (GV12).

3. Spleen and Stomach Deficiency

This group of patients most frequently has digestive system problems, such as indigestion, constipation, diarrhea or diarrhea alternating with constipation, nausea, no appetite, diarrhea after eating, gastric pain, weight loss, spontaneous sweat or night sweats, palpitations, tiredness or fatigue, peripheral neuropathy. The emotions found in this group often are in irritability and anxiety. Acupuncture should be given once or twice a week.

Pulse:
Slow, slippery; right *Guan* deep, left *Guan* thin and wiry.

Tongue:
Pale with teeth marks, large with white, thick or sticky coating on the spleen area.

Acupoints:
Taibai (Sp3), *Gongsun* (Sp4), *Shangqiu* (Sp5), *Sanyinjian* (SP6), *Shuifen* (CV9), *Zusanli* (S36), *Pishu*, (B20), *Weishu* (B21). With diarrhea, use: *Tienshu* (S25), *Baihui* (GV20). With neuropathy, use: *Bafang* (EX 69), *Yanlingqian* (G34), *Yinlingqian* (Sp9).

Auricular Points:
Spleen, Stomach, Endocrine, Heart.

Moxabustion:
Zusanli (S36), *Shenjue* (CV8).

4. Kidney Jin and Yin Deficiency

This group of patients most frequently has experienced weight loss, has a skin pallor, restless sleep with nightmares, night sweats, aching joints, lower back pain, tinnitus, sore throat, loss of balance, in women, irregular menstruation or dismenorrhea, in men, loss of sexual function and/or impotence. The emotions found in this group often include panic, fear and, in some instances, dementia.

Pulse:
Thin and deep, thready, especially in both Chi.

Tongue:
Red or purple, gray in patients with anemia, some cracks with thin coating or no coating at all and some thickness on the kidney area.

Acupoints:
Taixi (K4), *Senshu* (B23), *Zhishi* (B52), *Shenmen* (H7), *Sanyinjiao* (SP6).

With Lower back pain, use: *Dazui* (GV14), *Shenzhu* (GV12).

Auricular Points:
Kidney, Shenmen, Spleen, Endocrine.

Moxabustion:
Yongquan (K1), *Mingmen* (GV4).

5. Liver Yin Deficiency, Liver Qi Stagnation

Patients have or had different kinds of hepatitis, dry or bitter taste in the mouth, afternoon fever or feverish feeling, blurring of vision or burning feeling in eyes, dizziness, loss of appetite, abdominal distention, headache or migraine. The emotions found in this group often are anger, mood swings, nervousness and sensitivity.

Pulse:
Thin, fast, wiry, compared with left *Cun* pulse, the left *Guan* is tighter and bigger and sometimes weaker.

Tongue:
Red, dry, small, some purple spots with thin, yellow or thick, white, dry coating.

Acupoints:
Taichong (L3), *Neiguang* (P6), *Taixi* (K4), *Ganshu* (B18), *Dangshu* (U19), *Fuliu* (K7), *Hegu*, (L4).

Auricular Points:
Liver, Shenmen, Endocrine, Sympathetic.

Moxabustion:
Sanyinjiao (S6).

6. Yin and Yang Deficiency, Qi and Xue Stagnation

Most frequent symptoms include fatigue, dirty-like skin, chest or abdominal pain, shortness of breath, weight loss from wasting syndrome, cold intolerance, dizziness, tinnitus, palpitation, pale face and nails. This group is slower to respond emotionally, and often feels depressed. Acupuncture for this group should be given twice a week or more.

Pulse:
Deep, thin and very weak, thready.

Tongue:
Pale, dry or purple with spots and peeling, spotting coating.

Acupoints:
Shanzhong (CV1), *Qihai* (CV6), *Hegu* (L4), *Xuehai* (Sp10), *Baihui* (GV20),*Sanyinjiao* (SP6).

Auricular Points:
Kidney, Spleen, Endocrine, Adrenal Gland.

Moxabustion:
Guanyuan (CV4), *Bahui* (GV20).

Acupuncture Treatment for HIV Infection in the United States

From the beginning of the AIDS epidemic in the early 1980s, HIV-infected people and people with AIDS had already begun to utilize acupuncture treatment.

As a pioneer in the use of acupuncture treatment for HIV and AIDS, Lincoln Hospital Acupuncture Clinic in New York began treating a group of 200 AIDS patients with acupuncture and Chinese herbs from 1982 to 1987. Before AZT began to be widely used, there were positive treatment approaches and results at Lincoln.

Also in New York, the Gay Men's Health Crisis has been providing acupuncture to AIDS patients since 1989. Volunteer acupuncturists see 50 to 80 patients per week on a regular basis.

The Chicago AIDS Alternative Health Project was one of the first acupuncture clinics dedicated exclusively to the treatment of AIDS patients. It was founded in 1986. A report in 1987 of 16 patients who had previously been diagnosed with PCP (pneumocystis carinii pneumonia) revealed that there was considerable and prolonged relief from fatigue, shortness of breath and mucous discharge. Most patients gained weight and were able to return to work. In the same city in 1989, the North Side AIDS Project was founded and began to see AIDS patients and expand its services to become the largest AIDS clinic for alternative treatments in Chicago. The North Side AIDS Project currently has 30 volunteer acupuncturists, who see 200 HIV/AIDS patients six days per week.

In San Francisco, Quan Yin Acupuncture and Herb Center was one of the first centers to treat HIV patients with acupuncture and herbs. In 1986, it formed the Quan Yin Healing Arts Center. There, every week, over 200 HIV-infected people receive acupuncture, Chinese herbs, nutrition, yoga, massage, group therapy and visualization therapy and counseling. Quan Yin Healing Arts Center has pioneered an intensive training program for acupuncture and medical professionals in the use of acupuncture and herbs to treat persons with HIV infection.

In Massachusetts, the Somerville Acupuncture Center began to see HIV infected patients in 1984. In 1990, this experience spawned the AIDS Care Project in Boston, which has become one of the largest acupuncture treatment centers for HIV patients in the United States. By 1992, the project staff of 25 volunteer acupuncturists and 50 acupuncture assistants gave approximately 350 acupuncture treatments per month to 250 AIDS and ARC patients. In 1994, 15 acupuncturists and 35 interns give 500 acupuncture and herbal treatments per month.

In 1988, a group of volunteer physicians, acupuncturists, physical therapists and Chiropractors formed the Austin Immune Health Clinic to provide a variety of new alternative approaches for people with HIV infection. Later, the clinic became the HIV Wellness Center, where hundreds of patients have been treated since its inception.

Also in 1988, in Portland, Oregon, Hooper Center (a treatment center for people with substance abuse problems) started to give acupuncture treatments to HIV infected patients. The center grew into the Portland Addiction Acupuncture Center, where they continue to give acupuncture and Chinese herbal treatments to the clinic patients.

In 1989, Kang Wen Clinic opened in Seattle, Washington. This clinic began operations in partially donated space with donated work by acupuncturists. Although small in size, this clinic has done much to make acupuncture available to HIV-infected people who would ordinarily not have this kind of treatment available to them. Once a week, six volunteers give treatments to 30 patients.

In conjunction with the University of Miami in Miami, Florida, a group of acupuncturists volunteer their services to a group study of 40 AIDS patients using acupuncture and Chinese herbs. A nationally broadcast television report featured this study and how acupuncture and Chinese herbal treatments give long-term survivors an improved quality of life.

In 1990, the Immune Enhancement Center in San

Francisco, California, opened with Ryan White funding. This center's 10 volunteers give acupuncture, herbal and massage treatments to 180 patients per week.

More patients with HIV infection recognize the benefits of acupuncture and more reports about the positive results of acupuncture in treating HIV infection are being published. As a result, the Federal government has begun to fund programs that will allow more patients access to acupuncture treatment. In July 1992, the first Ryan White funding for acupuncture was given to the American College of Traditional Chinese Medicine in San Francisco. This College is now able to provide AIDS patients with acupuncture treatment and Chines herbs. As the Ryan White funding has been expanded to included other clinics in the United States, so has the expanded availability of acupuncture and Chinese herbs for the treatment of HIV infection.

The above information is only a partial list of United States clinics using acupuncture treatment for HIV infection. It is clear that there will be a marked increase in the demand for acupuncture treatment among HIV-infected patients. It confirms that acupuncture, one of the oldest medicines, is increasingly being utilized as a treatment for HIV infection. Equally important, the attitudes of Western medical practitioners toward acupuncture and Traditional Chinese Medicine are being revised.

For further information on acupuncture treatment locations, please review the listing at the end of this book and contact your local AIDS organizations.

Notes

1) J.Y. Liu. *Yuennan Magazine of Traditional Chinese Medicine*, 1990: 23-24 (1).

2) Y.M. Yang. *Acupuncture Research*, 1988: 63 (3).

3) R.X. Zhou. *Abstract of Symposium on Acupuncture and Immune Function*, 1988: 205.

4) L.N. Hu. *Jiangshu Magazine of Traditional Chinese Medicine*, 1990: 2.

5) M. Cui. *Magazine of Traditional Chinese Medicine*, 1990: 3.

6) K.J. Chen. *Henang Magazine of Traditional Chinese Medicine*, 1984: (4), (5).

7) Y.F. Qiu. *China Lab Immune Magazine*, 1990: 2 (1).

8) H.P. Chen. *Jiangshu Magazine of Traditional Chinese Medicine,* 1990.

9) M.O. Smith. "Results of Chinese Medical Treatment Show Frequent Symptom Relief and Some Apparent Long-Term Remissions," World Congress of Acupuncture and Natural Medicine, Beijing, 1987.

10) N. Rabinowitz. "Acupuncture and the AIDS Epidemic: Reflections on the Treatment of 200 Patients in Four Years," *American Journal of Acupuncture*, 1987:15, 35-42.

11) D.R. Cornblath and J. C. McArthur. "Predominantly Sensory Neuropathy in Patients with AIDS and AIDS-Related Complex," *Neurology*, 1988: 38, 794-796.

12) M. Goh. "Acupuncture Treatment for Neuropathy Patients with HIV Infection," 2nd World Federal Acupuncture Society Conference, Paris, 1990.

Shiatsu and HIV Infection

Introduction

There are many different forms and styles of Shiatsu in the United States today. Zen Shiatsu, Macrobiotic Shiatsu, Bare Foot Shiatsu and Five Element Shiatsu to name but a few. The techniques and methods may vary, but the underlying core of the work and theory is similar. This article describes Zen Shiatsu and Five Element Shiatsu.

Shiatsu offers a holistic approach to bodywork, taking into account what is happening with the client physically and emotionally as well as considering the impact of the environment. In a session, the Shiatsu practitioner does not give energy or take away problems but helps the client move towards a state of balance and harmony. If the body is balanced, the body is best able to heal itself.

Most forms of Shiatsu are done on a mat, with the

client fully clothed. Techniques used are a combination of stretches, range of motion, rocking and shaking movements, and pressure from fingers, hands, forearms, knees and feet. Shiatsu actually is a Japanese word meaning finger pressure.

Shiatsu is rooted in the same theory as acupuncture, which dates back to before 2600 years B.C. in China. When trade routes started opening up between China and Japan about 550 AD, Chinese monks brought this acupuncture theory and a type of bodywork to Japan called Amma. In the early 1900s, Shiatsu grew out of Amma and was developed and recognized by the Japanese government. In the 1960s, word of Shiatsu started spreading to the United States and the rest of the world.

Pathways and Energy: Meridians and Ki

Shiatsu deals with pathways of energy, called meridians. These meridians run throughout the body and regulate all body systems, both physical and emotional. Along these meridians flows a vital life force, an energy called Ki (Chi or Qi). The flow of Ki should be even and unobstructed for balance and harmony to be maintained in the body.

There are 12 meridians that correspond to organs, organ function, and also to emotional characteristics. For example, there are the Lung, Heart, Stomach and Gall Bladder meridians, with each meridian relating to specific emotions such as grief, joy, worry and anger. Along these meridians are points, called tsubos. Tsubos are where the energy is more active and tends to pool. These are the points where an acupuncturist would insert needles during treatment to tonify or sedate the energy. The Shiatsu practitioner, however, uses pressure on the tsubos, or works at stretching the body along the meridians to help facilitate energy flow.

When energy is flowing freely and organs are strong and functioning well, there is an energetic balance and one is said to be in harmony. In this state of harmony, the body works most efficiently and is best able to heal itself. Disharmonies or physical symptoms can develop when the Ki is not flowing smoothly. The internal and external environment as well as everything thought and felt affects this flow of energy. The Shiatsu practitioner tries to help the client come into a more balanced state by working on the extremes in energy flow. An area that is weak, depleted or low in energy it would be said to be Kyo. A Shiatsu practitioner would attempt to tonify this area to move the body closer to its natural state of balance. The other extreme would be an area that is very full, active or excessive. This area would be called Jitsu, and a Shiatsu practitioner would try to sedate or disperse that energy. Then, if the energy is flowing smoothly, the body is best able to do whatever it needs to do.

Large Intestine Meridian

Although it is labeled with a specific organ, the Large Intestine meridian is associated with much more than the organ and its function in Western thought. In Shiatsu, the Large Intestine meridian's main function is elimination. The pathway holds the energy that supports this function on a physical and emotional level. Physically, there are many ways the body can eliminate: through the bowels, skin, nose and breath, through coughing, sneezing, exhaling and defecating. All these activities are related to the Large Intestine meridian. If there is an imbalance in the energy along the meridian, problems may occur with these functions. Symptoms could appear as overactive elimination or the opposite, extreme holding on. In the bowels, these extremes could be diarrhea or constipation. In the case of the nose, the extremes of a runny nose (elimination) or congested sinuses (holding on) could occur.

The Body Is Not Separate from the Mind and Emotions.

Emotional functions mirror physical functions. Emotionally, people can hold onto material things, habits or friends and can also let them go. Someone who is described in psychological terms as being "anal retentive" finds it difficult to let go of details, habits and emotions. This individual also could be showing this holding onto imbalance. Someone who is a pack rat, who collects and holds onto every magazine, piece of paper, rubber band, letter and souvenir, may begin to fill up the living space until the living environment is very full (constipated or congested). This may be indicating an imbalance in the smooth flow of being able to take in and then eliminate. The opposite might be someone who eliminates things as soon as they enter the life or living space. This person may not be very open and may live in a very spare and simple way, perhaps distancing himself or herself from others.

The emotion that is directly associated with the Large Intestine meridian is grief. Grief or the grieving process occurs when something or someone in life that has been lost (eliminated) and we are not ready to let go of that something or someone. The grieving process continues until we finally are able to let go. Grief is very much concerned with elimination and letting go of people and things. It is therefore connected to Large Intestine energy.

Shiatsu theory teaches that how we respond

emotionally affects us physically. It might not be obvious at first. It could be as subtle as a shift in breathing and muscle tension. Inversely, physical things can also effect emotions. For example, having diarrhea could make the individual feel less outgoing and more self conscious and shy. The stronger the physical or emotional upset and the longer its duration the more likely symptoms will arise and intensify, become more apparent and cross the mind-body barrier.

Grieving the loss of a favorite hat could effect a minor change in the energy flow. It may effect how and what the individual is doing but it will probably pass quickly with balance soon being restored. The loss of a significant person in life often creates a larger imbalance, which will influence emotional and physical balance for a longer period of time. The natural tendency would be to cry and possibly sob. The chest may heave as deep breaths are taken in and let go. Blowing the nose is part of this elimination process. Trying to shut off grieving before it has been finished may result in physical symptoms resembling the grieving process, such as a cold. With a cold, the chest may heave with coughing, eyes may tear and there is a runny nose and a need to blow the nose.

The Five Element Theory

The Chinese observed their environment and discovered basic elements which had specific characteristics and interrelationships. They assumed that these elements and relationships were also happening within ourselves. This is the concept of "macro equals micro." The solar system is made of the same things and has the same inner workings and interrelationships as the Earth, which also is reflected in ourselves. In the world around us there is Metal,

Earth, Water, Fire and Wood. So, the "Five Element Theory" follows that these elements, their qualities and interrelationships are also within ourselves.

Water

In the environment there is Water. It can be calm like a lake or powerful like a waterfall. It flows like a river and has cycles like the tides of an ocean. These characteristics of water are also found within us. We can be calm or powerful. Our bodies have cycles and rhythms and we can let our emotions flow or damn them up. In Oriental theory, these emotional characteristics would be Water energy within us and would be described in these Water element terms.

Fire

Around us in our environment is Fire. There is the warmth of the sun and the fire we use to cook. A flame is dynamic and lively, it radiates warmth and energy. We also possess these qualities. Someone with excess Fire energy might be someone full of spark, lively, enthusiastic, someone "all fired up." Someone who radiates great warmth emotionally or someone who is be running a fever might also be someone with excess Fire energy. Someone could indicate a lack of Fire energy by feeling cold, not being warm emotionally, "frigid" sexually, or "burnt out." Either extreme is an imbalance which could lead to, or be the cause of lack of Fire.

Earth and Wood

The Earth element is related to feeling grounded and centered, connected to the earth. It has to do with fertility like the Mother Earth. The Wood element within us is like the energy of a tree, being rooted and reaching for the sky with a strong trunk and flexibility to bend in the breeze. The Wood element is the ability to be flexible yet strong both physically and emotionally.

Metal

Besides physical and emotional situations effecting our health, the balance of an element in our environment can also be a major influence. A certain amount of an element can aid its corresponding functioning, but too much or too little can lead to an imbalance. For example dryness can effect the Metal element. A little dryness can aid the function of the Metal element and the Large Intestine meridian, but any extreme could interfere with that function. So the dryness of the air can effect breathing, skin and even emotions. This can be illustrated by dry air and heat in the winter, which often contribute to respiratory problems like colds and flu.

Yin and Yang

The theory surrounding opposite characteristics contained within a whole is known as the Yin/Yang theory. Everything contains an ebb and flow of Yin and Yang. These polarities act as complements. The Chinese character or pictogram for Yang shows a sunny side of a hill. The sunny side is lighter, warmer and more active than the shady side. The shady side of the hill in the pictogram is Yin. Yin is quieter, darker, less active than Yang.

Everything can be divided into this Yin/Yang coupling. A day can be divided into daytime (more Yang) and night-time (more Yin). The twelve traditional meridians are divided into the Five Elements with the elements then being paired in a Yin/Yang partnership.

The Large Intestine meridian (Yang) is paired with the Lung meridian (Yin) within the Metal element. The major function of the Lung meridian is intake, which is a complement to the large Intestine function of elimination. The Stomach meridian (Yang) is coupled with the Spleen meridian (Yin) for Earth, the Bladder meridian (Yang) with the Kidney meridian (Yin) for Water, the Small Intestine meridian (Yang) with the Heart meridian (Yin) for Absolute Fire, the Triple Heater meridian (Yang) with the Pericardium meridian (Yin) for Supplemental Fire, and Gall Bladder (Yang) is paired with the Liver meridian (Yin) for Wood.

HIV: A Pattern of Disharmony

Shiatsu practitioners look for corresponding signs and symptoms that may indicate a pattern of disharmony of Yin/Yang. They may look at skin color, the way one moves and talks. They may inquire about how one is doing emotionally and if there has been any recent changes in life physically, emotionally or environmentally. When they touch the body, they are still looking for imbalances by palpating for Kyo or Jitsu areas along the meridians.

The range of symptoms and emotions that arise with HIV-related illness are great. Each person is very unique and the energy and balance for each person often changes from moment to moment. Thus there are a very few specific imbalances that everyone dealing with HIV would be treated for. Each case would be looked at separately. However, people tend to have chronic imbalances even before HIV. They have developed and learned imbalances throughout life. When an extreme situation like AIDS arises, the disharmonies in a person may be exaggerated, leading to more pronounced symptoms and thus perhaps an easier evaluation of their imbalances.

One meridian that is important in treating HIV is the Triple Heater meridian. The body's immune system is very much tied to the function of this meridian. The Triple Heater regulates body temperature and the energy that allows the body to run a fever to fight off disease. This energy is commonly strained in HIV. For example, if this energy is not strong, the body may run a low-grade fever for a long time, unable to rise sufficiently to deal with the problem.

People living in the HIV+ community or having contact with others dealing with AIDS usually experience grief. They may be dealing with loss of friends as well as the loss of function and are grieving over their own life. Often, this could contribute to an imbalance in the Metal element. So, colds, skin problems and even pneumonia may show up, which could partly be caused by these imbalances in Metal.

Many emotions may come up for someone with HIV such as anger, frustration, worry and depression. Although these are emotions everyone has at some point, they often could be stronger due to the situation of HIV infection or AIDS. Thus, there is more likelihood that these emotions may have an impact on physical health. The treatment is not to restrict or limit these emotions but to let them flow more freely and move to a more balanced state. Any time we restrict or force, we are constraining the natural flow of our energy.

A Shiatsu practitioner locates where physical and emotional holding occurs in the body and encourages and supports the energy to flow in a more balanced, efficient way, thus maximizing the potential energy in the entire body. Many clients feel like they have more energy to use after a session. A practitioner can also point out environmental influences that could be putting a strain on health.

The Shiatsu practitioner does not give energy to the client or take energy away. The practitioner simply facilitates the client coming back to a natural balance. If the body is in balance the body can then best heal itself.

Massage Protocol To Treat HIV/AIDS

Benefits of Massage

Massage is one form of treatment that is available to every Person With AIDS and HIV-positive individual. It can be given by a massage therapist or a friend. The massage techniques described in this article can be used as a massage protocol at home or in a clinical setting.

Most everyone enjoys a good massage. The overall effect of massage is a feeling of being more relaxed than before the treatment. But, what are some of the other effects of massage?

Massage affects body, mind and spirit. Like other alternative treatments, it embraces the full spectrum of philosophical approaches to healing found in holistic, classical Eastern and some Western schools of thought. Most modalities, whether they are Eastern or Western, employ techniques that ultimately affect the body in similar ways.

One effect that appears to occur with massage is to return the body to a state of balance, where fluids and energy are unblocked and flowing more freely. This also is a part of the process in which the body begins to heal itself. Within the context of Western physiology, this reaction is induced by stimulating the return of both venous Blood and lymph through their vessels back to the Heart and by increasing the flow of arterial Blood to areas of treatment. This flow of Blood is important in maintaining a healthy internal environment. Arterial Blood carries nutrients to each cell and venous Blood and lymph carries away cellular waste and toxic by-products of stress, abuse, disease, diet and drugs.

Many Eastern and some Western health care practitioners view disease as the result of an increasingly inhospitable and toxic internal environment. The accumulation of toxins in the body plays an important role in the progression of illness. Symptoms of disease are often the body's healthy response to a toxic environment. It is the body's attempt to throw off poisons in order to return to homeostasis or health. Physical or emotional abuses and foods that cannot be absorbed by our systems often result in putrefaction in the gut and production of toxins. Drugs with harmful side-effects also contribute to the gradual poisoning of the body and place additional stress on individual cells.

As more toxins are created or introduced into the body, the body's systems are placed under more stress and have a greater need to eliminate these toxins. A healthy body will filter and eliminate these toxins or poisons from the Blood and lymph systems through normal physical activity. But, when there is a progression of disease in the body, the Blood and lymph systems become over-stressed. They slow down as the disease progresses and the entire body is affected. Toxins begin to accumulate within cells, which soon become deprived of oxygen. Before long, tissues and organs cannot function at their optimum efficiency.

Massage cannot duplicate the role physical activity plays in maintaining the flow of lymph and venous Blood. But, massage can enhance diminished flow so that these fluids continue to be filtered and cleansed of poisons during circulation. Certain massage techniques will specifically aid the body in its elimination of toxins. Friction techniques create heat on the surface of the body, inducing perspiration and the elimination of toxins through the skin. Connective tissue massage and deep muscle techniques work to clear the connective tissues of toxic material, allowing toxins to surface from deeper layers of the body.

When applied to specific areas of tissues and organs, massage brings Blood and hence more oxygen to those areas that may not be getting the oxygen they need to work at optimum levels. Massage to the Liver can foment hepatic activity, prompting that organ in its function of transforming toxins into less poisonous forms, which can then be eliminated by the Kidneys. Abdominal massage has been shown to stimulate activity in the Kidneys and to promote urination. In addition, massage to the Abdomen can ease the passage of food from the Stomach to the Intestines and stimulate peristalsis, which aids the process of food absorption and elimination.

Because massage can assist in elimination, it may be helpful as part of a healing strategy for HIV and AIDS. Currently, many drugs taken for HIV or AIDS are accompanied by toxic side-effects. Aiding the body in its efforts to filter and cleanse, regular massage treatments may delay or moderate some of those toxic effects. Massage techniques for the Liver and Kidneys may be of particular use to those who have chosen to combine alternative therapies with standard Western treatment therapies. By providing the body with more oxygen and nourishment, massage helps the body to continue to work as efficiently as possible for as long as possible.

Massage has several positive mechanical effects on the body. But, massage may affect the body in other, more subtle ways. One of the most important effects which massage appears to have is on the immune system.

Massage is touch. With we touch, we can communicate love, concern and compassion. Touch is an act of healing. Although we don't clearly understand why, scientific evidence has repeatedly shown that touch can influence the body to process disease in ways which are self-healing. Studies show that when touch is included as part of a treatment strategy, living beings are better able to transform otherwise harmful stimuli in ways that are healing to the body.

Love heals. When we communicate that love through touch, we open doors to healing. Massage allows the body to feel good. During periods of long illness, massage can reunite body and mind, so that the body is not perceived as the enemy. Bernie Siegel recommends massage to his patients on the morning of chemotherapy treatments. These patients go into treatments feeling at peace and report fewer side-effects after the treatments

Touch also can unlock and transform emotions, drawing feelings to the surface and unlocking them.

This effect of touch can create and an acceptance of locked up emotions, enable dignity, control and peace to what at times can be a difficult journey.

Oriental medicine provides another understanding of energy as it circulates dynamically throughout the human body in its own energetic pathways. These pathways also link together all of the body's tissues and organs and provide a pathway to diagnose and interpret changes in the body before they are manifested physically. A basic premise of "dis-ease" of the body, mind or spirit is that before physical symptoms appear, there is an abnormality in the balance and circulation of energy. This imbalance, if not corrected, leads to organ and system malfunction and degeneration. The best way to heal the body is to adjust and balance its energy flow before there is any physical damage. Once a physical problem does manifest, correcting energy disturbances may allow the body to begin to heal itself. Chinese massage, Jin Shin Do and Shiatsu, work to release any blockages or stasis in the body by effecting changes within its energetic patterns, and to balance and restore the body's natural flow of energy.

Massage, when combined with acupuncture, Chinese herbal therapy, Qi Gong and food therapy, seems to have had a positive affect on the overall state of health in patients with HIV/AIDS. This combination also appears to ease and to delay some of the more toxic effects of Western drugs prescribed by Western medical practitioners for HIV infection and AIDS. The treatment also seems to relieve or diminish some of the physical symptoms associated with HIV and AIDS. Just as important, it can contribute toward restoring a measure of serenity or emotional balance.

Chinese Massage Protocol for HIV/AIDS

This massage protocol is based on the principles of Chinese medicine. It was developed by Jeffrey C. Yuen as a treatment for HIV and has been incorporated by an AIDS clinic in New York City for the past two years as part of the overall treatment plan.

The massage is based upon the premise that in HIV infection, special energetic channels (the Divergents), which are conduits for vital energies in the body, have been weakened by lifestyle stresses, including sexual and drug abuse. Abuse is a relative term here, and it may be different for everyone. These channels serve as communication between the deep interior and surface of the body. The energy becomes increasingly unable to reach either the surface, to protect the body from external pathogens, or to the deepest layers of the interior.

This energy, which is housed in the Kidneys, serves as the fundamental source of all of the body's energetic requirements. When the immune functions are weakened, less of this energy is available to tissues and organs to perform their functions. The Liver becomes congested and unable to clean and filter the toxic by-products of food, air, drugs and other stressors. Toxins begin to accumulate in the body and the terrain becomes ripe for the growth of opportunistic infections.

This massage treatment protocol is designed to free up this trapped vital energy (Wei). When Wei is available to return to the surface of the body, it helps the body to fight against pathogens and to direct energy back to the Kidneys.

In Chinese medicine, the Kidneys are called the

"Root of Life," precisely because they store this vital energy (Qi) and make it available to all of our other organs and tissues. Indirectly, this massage treatment protocol nourishes not only Kidneys but all tissues and organs. In addition, the massage stimulates the flow of Blood and promotes lymphatic drainage, encouraging the release of toxins in the body. Finally, the basic premise of Chinese medicine is that by directing energy to the right places in the body, it will be able to use that energy to heal itself. By bringing the body's energy and the mind's attention to each area as it is touched, the massage also serves as a tool for self-healing.

What can be expected from this massage treatment? Some people may feel energized after the treatment or a little tired, as energy moves inward to nourish the Kidneys. Either reaction is fine. People who are generally asymptomatic HIV+ may feel some symptoms (headaches, colds, low-grade fevers, bitter taste in the mouth, slight muscular pain and/or emotional release). These symptoms are a result of the body's release of toxins or trapped energy that has been released by the massage. Again, these reactions are fine. They are a sign of healing and, in fact, of the body's health. Some people also report feeling more centered, less irritable and generally "better." This feeling lasts one day to one week after the massage.

Precautions

As with all massage treatments, common sense precautions are necessary:

1) Be careful of hygiene, work carefully around fragile areas, don't touch anything on the skin which may be communicable and don't work on top of lesions.

2) Don't do the massage if you or your massage partner suspect an infectious condition such as herpes or tuberculosis.

3) In general, before receiving the treatment, check with a medical doctor or health practitioner, particularly if you have a very weakened or weakening condition. This massage should not adversely affect but may help conditions such as KS, PCP, CMV and cancer. Some doctors advise against massage therapy for cancer patients although this view is not uniformly held. Any specific condition should be discussed with the attending physician.

4) This protocol is not appropriate for someone with a kidney infection.

General Instructions / Directions

As you work with a partner, your primary aim is to free energy that is trapped in the body and direct that energy to the Kidneys. The first set of diagrams (pages 94-95) map out the general course and direction of the protocol. The second set of diagrams (pages 102-103) indicate the specific areas of massage.

In the first set of diagrams (pages 94-95), begin by moving energy in the arms from the wrists to the shoulders (#1), and from the neck in front of the body to the collarbone (#2). Next, direct this energy as well as any energy trapped between the ribs first out to the sides of the body (#3), then, when your partner turns over, around the back to the spine and down to the Kidneys (#4 and #5).

After these moves, carefully free energy trapped around the upper vertebrae of the neck (#6) and the sacrum (#7), moving that energy toward the center of the body. Turn your partner over again and stimulate the Colon, following its ascending, transverse and descending parts (#8), and bringing that energy around once more toward the spine in back and the Kidneys (#9).

Finally, connect the spine to the front mid-line of the body by directing energy from the spine down through the sacrum into the tailbone (#10) and by shaking out the legs from the ankle to the hips.

As you read through the treatment protocol and review pages 102-103, do not worry if it seems complicated to you. In fact, keep it simple. Your intent essentially is to get energy flowing and moving within the body. The body itself will direct that energy where it needs it to go. Don't struggle with the moves. If the directions seem unclear to you, try to follow the intention and direction of each of the moves and create your own moves, which seem to accomplish that intent. Remember that intention and intuition play a very strong part in massage. You've known how to touch since you were born, and you already possess the intuition and the ability to touch someone in a healing way.

Please move gently through this massage. Try to move energy by focusing your attention on that area, by intention rather than brute strength. Essentially, you are prompting the body to make its own adjustments, not trying to mechanically force any changes. The numbers in parentheses contain the specific point designations for those who arer familiar with Oriental point locations.

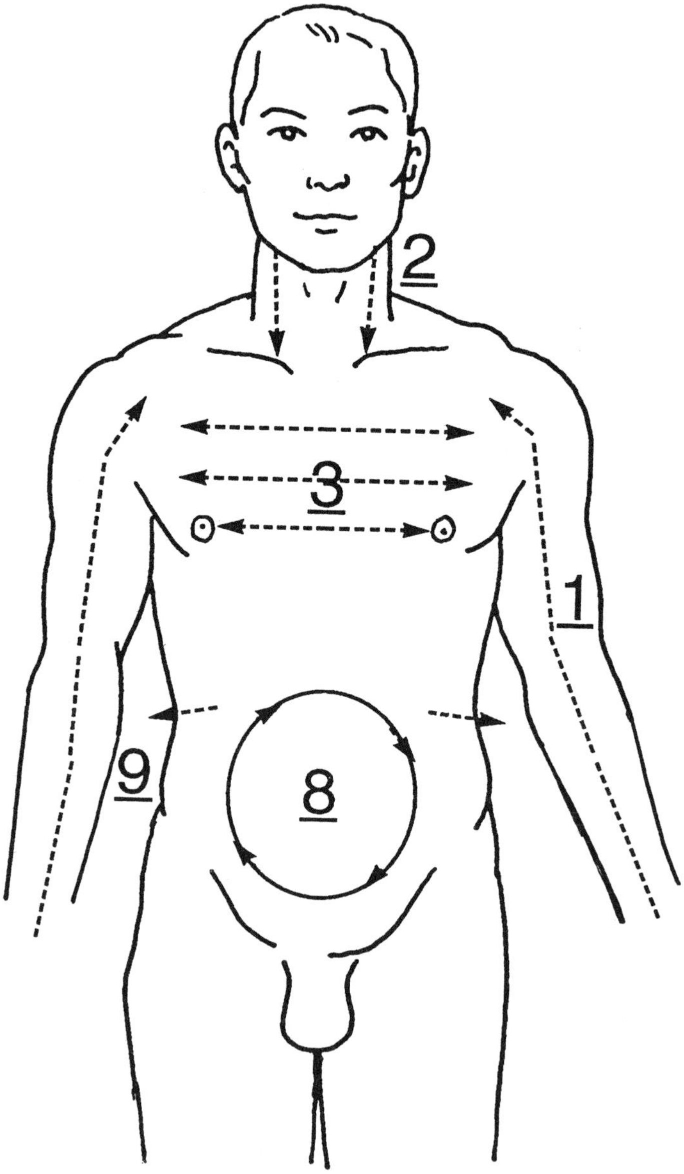
2
3
1
9
8

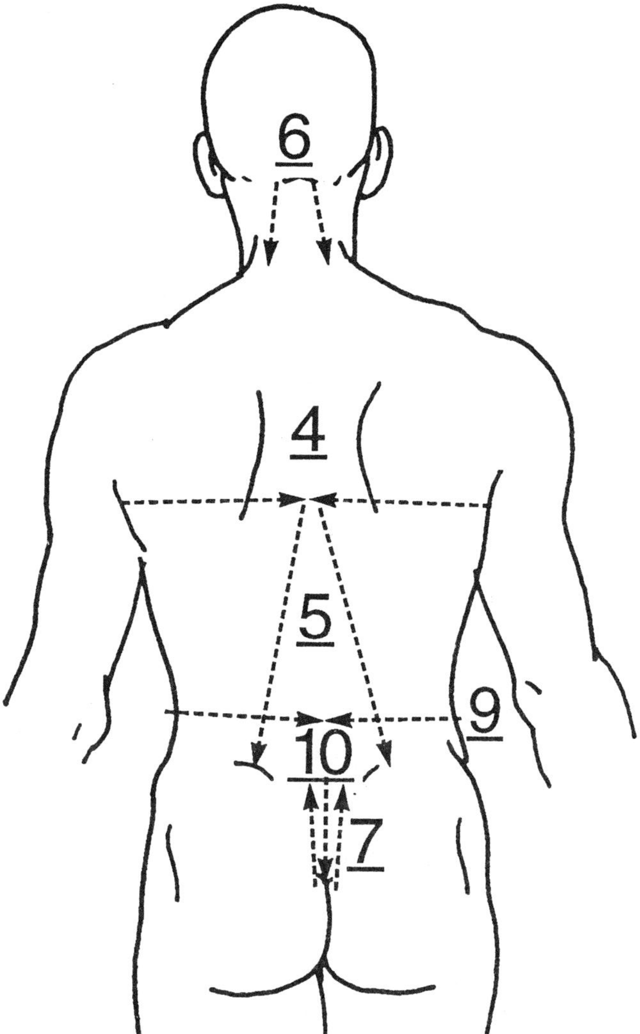
6
4
5
9
10
7

HIV Massage Protocol

Follow the diagrams for each specific move.

Your partner lies on his/her back:

1) **wrist:** Holding your partner's arm with one hand, rotate her writs with your other hand by grasping and rotating her middle finger in a circle. Rotate the wrist in both directions. (Note: always start with the middle finger.) Rotate each finger in both directions. *Intention: You are opening up the joint to release any energy that may be trapped and prompting the energy to begin to flow through energetic channels from the surface of the body to its interior. Surface energy gathers at the joints, and it is this energy that you are trying to free.*

2) **wrist, elbow, shoulder:** Holding the palm of her hand with both of your hands, shake her arm by vibrating the arm from the wrist to the shoulder. *Intention: same as above.*

3) **shoulder:** Rotate each shoulder in both directions while grasping the middle of the palm of the hand. *Intention: same as above.*

Repeat these first three moves for the other arm.

5) **neck:** Glide very gently along the carotid artery or the front muscles of the neck with your fingertips from behind the ear to the center of the collar bone. (ST12) *Intention: In this move, by moving energy on the upper part of the body, you will establish a connection with the lower body, specifically with the Kidneys according to a principle of Chinese medicine, which postulates, "as above, so below." This move actually prompts the body to re-establish*

the balance between the thyroid gland or "fire" above and the Kidneys or "water" below.

5) **middle of the collar bone, above the bone:** Gently tap or vibrate one fingertip into this point (ST12), located above and in the center of the collar bone. This is the point at which you ended in the previous move. *Intention: By gently tapping this point, you are prompting energy from the surface of the body to move through channels into the deepest energetic layer of the body, home of the Kidneys. You are also guiding lymph into its vessels. This point serves as a "waste receptacle," and its activation encourages the body to begin to dump its toxins out through appropriate channels.*

6) **interior end of the collar bone:** Make circular rotations in both directions with your fingertip at this point (ST11). *Intention: Here you simply want to activate this point, which directly affects the level of energy available to the body.*

7) **intercostal spaces between each rib from collar bone to level of nipples:** Using moderate pressure, glide your thumb or fingertips horizontally in the space between each rib, moving from the center breastbone outward toward the side of the body. Note: After avoiding tender breast tissue, be sure to continue on the outside of the breast to the side of the body. *Intention: With this move, you are trying to free up any energy that may be trapped between the ribs and bring that energy to the sides of the body. Soon, you will bring it to the back toward the spine in order that it may be used by the body's deepest energetic layers. By working in this area, (location of the Thoracic and Right Lymphatic Ducts), you are also facilitating the movement of lymph through its vessels.*

8) **point directly between the breasts at the level of the nipples:** Make circular rotations with your palm or fingertips going in both directions at this point (CV17). Note: Try to be sensitive to the amount of pressure required here. This area is not only physically sensitive, but it is an emotionally vulnerable spot, which is related to the energy of the Heart. Working here may elicit an emotional response as your partner releases the energy of a "Heart-ache," which she may have suppressed. *Intention: In Chinese medicine, this point is where all energy on the surface of the body eventually returns. By activating this point, you are prompting this energy to go inward and communicate with the Kidneys, home of our deepest energetic resources. You are encouraging the Kidneys to "rest and recuperate," to gather their energetic resources so that they will be available as the body needs them.*

Your partner turns over, lying on the stomach.

9) **axilla (armpit) to spine:** Glide your fingers from the area under the armpits on the sides of the body over the shoulder blades to the spine, "drawing" a horizontal line connecting the sides of the body to the spine. *Intention: By continuing on the back the "line" that you previously made through the ribs, you are bringing the energy that you freed on the front of the body to the spine. You also are freeing energy trapped in this area of the back. This movement prompts the body to begin draining toxins in the lymph fluid, which should be flowing more freely after your work on the front.*

10) **spine at the point of your imaginary line:** With the palm of your hand, make circular rotations in both directions at this point (GV9) located at the middle of your line in #9, between thoracic

vertebrae 7 and 8. (This point actually is located at the spine, level with the lower ends of the shoulder blades.) *Intention: Here you are stimulating the Diaphragm, which in Chinese medicine is the bridge linking the energy on the surface of the body with its more substantiated form of Blood. In other words, with this move, you are prompting energy to enter the level of Blood to nourish the internal organs and aid the body in filtering toxins. You have at this point in the massage directed energy to assist both the Blood and lymph in their efforts to cleanse and heal the body.*

11) **spine to waist:** Grasp your partner's waist at the level of the navel with both hands, thumbs on the back of the body. Note the point (BL23) at which your thumbs fall. Now draw another line connecting the spinal point above in #10 to these two points on either side of your partner's waist. Sometimes, it is easiest to do this gently with the crook of your elbow. *Intention: In this move, you are now directing the energy that you previously freed from the spine into the Kidneys, which are "resting" and ready to receive it.*

12) **waist:** Make circular rotations in each direction with your thumbs at the above point on either side of your partner's waist (BL23). *Intention: With this move, you are encouraging the Kidneys to regulate the amount of toxins being stored or released from the body.*

13) **neck:** With your partner's forehead lying directly on the table (neck straight), gently glide your fingertips down her neck from the ear to the spine, stopping at the point on the spine that is approximately level with the height of the shoulders. The correct spinal point (GV14) is

located under the first large vertebrae you feel. *Intention: Essentially, the same as for move #4 for the front of the neck. You are trying to mobilize surface energies and direct them to this important spinal point (GV14).*

14) neck: Now "knead" this area along the sides of the vertebrae from the occiput (ridge) of the skull to the previous spinal point. *Intention: You are trying to free up energy that is commonly trapped in this area and direct it into this point.*

15) spinal point (GV14): Make circular rotations in both directions with the palm of your hands at the above point. *Intention: Now that you have directed energy to this point, you must activate it, so that it will send energy inward.*

Note: For the next step, your partner should keep her chin on the table, in order to close off the neck. If not, the energy you free may travel up to the head and cause a headache.

16) sacrum: Try to knead this area from the bottom of the sacrum moving up to the top, approximately level with the waist. *Intention: To free energy commonly trapped here and direct it into another very important point in Chinese medicine (GV4), which encourages the Kidneys to "bank" or store more of our vital energy.*

Your partner turns over, lying once again on her back.

17) Colon: Apply perpendicular pressure with your fingertips along the ascending, transverse and descending Colon. Work up the right side of your partner first, starting below the navel and working up almost to the rib cage, then work across and down the left side. As you apply pressure to the Colon, your partner breathes into her abdomen, trying to lift your fingers. After each breath, push a little deeper. **Note: If your partner feels any sharp pains in the abdomen, lighten your pressure.** Continue at each position until your partner can lift your hand and you feel a pulse with your fingertips. Repeat exercise with fingertips moving in diagonally toward the center of the body. *Intention: Here you are stimulating the movement of Blood through the aorta, the major vessel transporting Blood from the Heart to the rest of the body. You also are prompting the body to direct energy from its surface into the Blood, once again stimulating the Blood to cleanse and nourish the organs and tissues of the body. The exercise will also encourage the movement of food through the Colon, prompting better elimination. By repeating the exercise with diagonal movements, you are stimulating and regulating (Chung Mai) energy at the deepest layers of the body.*

Your partner turns over on her stomach once again.

18) ribs on the back: Find the lowest rib on the back of the body and gently "rake" your fingers from the side of this rib toward the spine at the level of the waist (GV4). **Please be careful at this fragile rib.** *Intention: With this move, you are prompting the channels that house our deepest constitutional energy to begin to regulate that energy according to the body's needs.*

19) sacrum and coccyx: Using moderately deep pressure, move from the waist toward the end of the tailbone on the mid-line of the body (GV4-GV1).

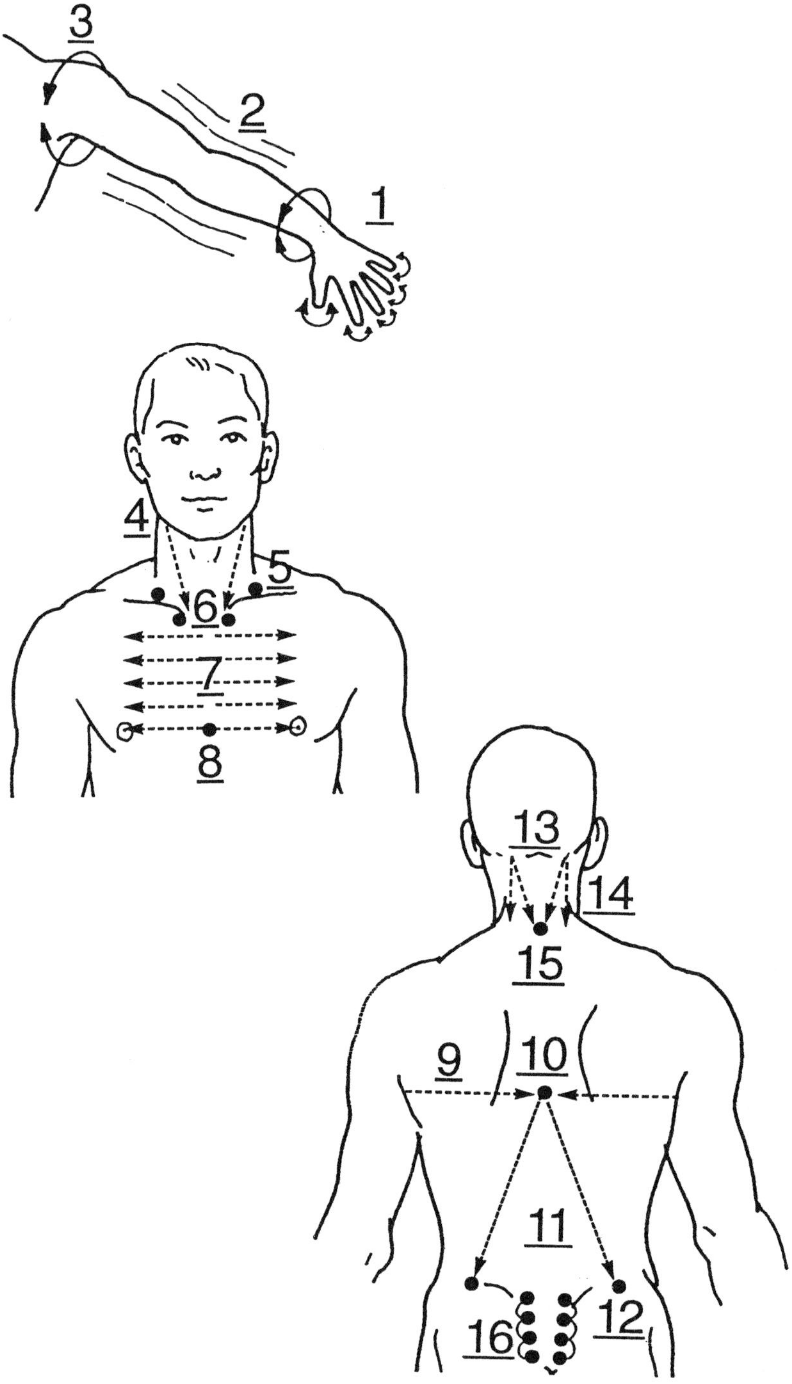
3
2
1
4
5
6
7
8
13
14
15
9
10
11
12
16

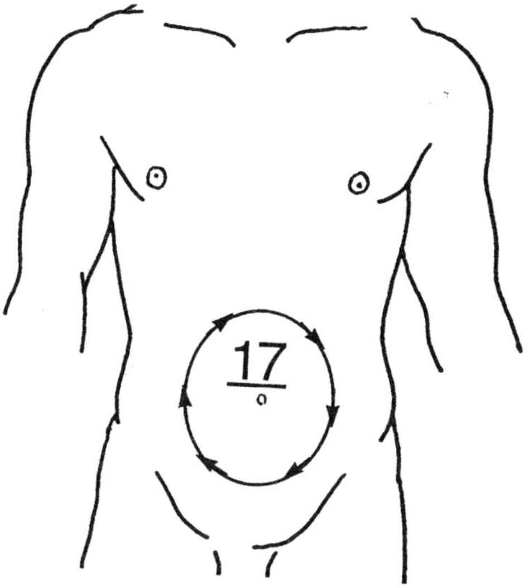
17

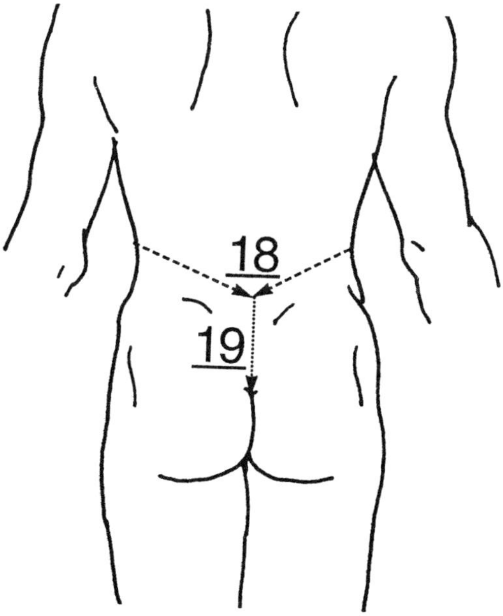
18
19

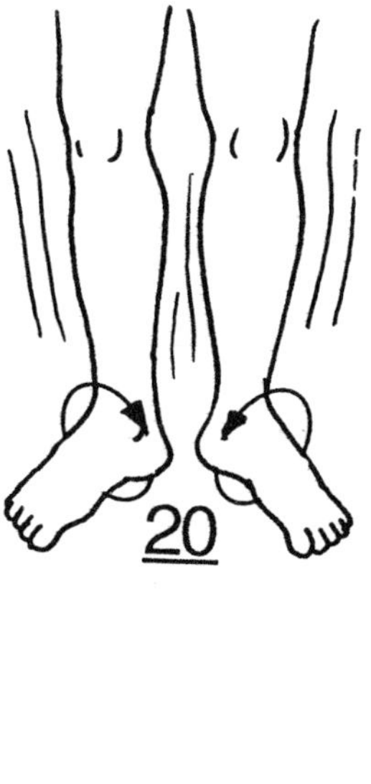
20

Intention: To encourage energy to move from spine to front of the body, completing this "energetic tour" and putting back into natural circulation any trapped energy that you have liberated.

Your partner turns over for the last time to lie on her back.

20) ankles: Supporting your partner's foot with one hand on the leg, rotate the ankle inward. Then, holding her leg with both of your hands, shake the leg, trying to vibrate into the thigh. Repeat on the other side. *Intention: as above.*

Congratulations! You have finished.

Final Thoughts

There are a number of other massage techniques that you might use. But, far more important than any technique is the opportunity that massage offers for the communication of unconditional love and compassion through touch in the care of human beings. Use this protocol as a tool, but use your love and compassion to heal.

The technique is only a vehicle to say with your Heart what you may not be able to say with your voice. Watching a loved one go through the process of disease can be a long and very hard road. It is not always possible to find the right words to communicate all that one is feeling. But, therapeutic massage requires no words, simply touch, offered unconditionally, which allows the body to go in whatever direction necessary on its road to self-healing.

The gift of massage is its ability to bring someone back to a quiet space within him or herself beyond the turmoil of emotions and pain. This is a place of strength, where we can return again and again. This is the place of real healing. To give someone access to that place, even for a few minutes, is no small gift.

The Influence of Qi Gong on the Immune System

Qi Gong, also called Chi Gong, is a form of Chinese exercise that involves: 1) posture, 2) breathing regulation, and 3) brain tranquilizing.

Many papers have reported on the results of Chinese experiments on the effects of Qi Gong on the immune system. The results of these experiments were selected from international journals and publications from 1984-1989.

Several of the experiments that have been published report on the favorable effects of Qi Gong through its stimulation of the immune system. I have excluded the most numerous papers that report on cancer patients who submit to personal training in Qi Gong and those papers which investigate cancer patients who have undergone treatment with Wai Qi. The clinical results of the therapeutic effects of Qi Gong on cancer is a subject area which deserves special attention. Also excluded are the accounts of the observations of medical staff members or of the accounts of patients who have healed themselves, which have appeared in popular Qi Gong journals in China.

Twenty-two articles that discuss the principal effects of Qi Gong on immunity have been selected. They are divided into three categories:

1) the *in vitro* effects of Wai Qi (projection of energy from the hand);

2) the effects of Wai Qi on living creatures (laboratory rats and cancer patients; and

4) the effects of Qi Gong exercises on immunity.

In Vitro Effects of Wai Qi

Wai Qi is the energy of the body emitted by Qi Gong experts. The majority of these practitioners emit the energy from the hand or from the Tian Mu "Eye of Heaven" point. The "Eye of Heaven" point, called Yin Tang in Chinese acupuncture, corresponds with the "Third Eye" in Indian Yoga teaching, and is located on the forehead between the eyebrows.

Qi Gong experts are selected according to their experience and, in most of the literature, they have been screened in advance for the power of the emission of their Qi by electromagnetic, infra-red or random laser measurements.

Ye Ming and Shen Jiagi (1) of Shanghai conducted trials on the comparative influence of Wai Qi from a Qi Gong expert (subject A), a long-term practitioner (subject B), and a lay person (subject C) on a culture of human lymphocytes. A total of 420 samples were analyzed according to four criteria:

1) absolute number of surviving lymphocytes;

2) power of lymphoblastic transformation;

3) percentage of Et RFC and Ea RFC;

4) synthesis of lymphocytic ADN.

The three participants had been asked to emit a "vital Qi" and then a "deadly Qi." The results of "deadly Qi" did not show any power of destruction of normal lymphocytes, with 98 percent surviving. But, in "vital Qi" emissions, 82 percent of the behaviors of the lymphocytes and the membrane receptors were influenced (grew) with subject A, 70 percent with subject B, and 0 percent with subject C.

The authors were able to show that under the influence of "vital Qi," the synthesis of lymphocytic ADN was increased, but that it also decreased under the influence of "deadly Qi."

Bi Aihua, et. al., of the Medical University of Tongji (2) analyzed 13 samples of blood from healthy donors divided into two groups: one group serving as a control, thus creating a total of 26 samples.

The lymphocytic power was studied under the influence of Wai Qi from two Qi Gong experts. The results showed a significant increase (p 0.01, p 0.01, p 0.05) respectively for parameters Tac+, Dq+ and DR+ in the treated specimens compared with the controls.

Hu Zong Lian, et. al., of the Anti-Cancer Research Center of Hospital 81 of Nanking (3) showed a significant influence of Wai Qi on the terminal granulocytic differentiation of HL-60 cells of promyelocytic leukemia in comparison with a control.

Guan Hao Ben and Yan Jin Hing of Canton (4) showed an influence of Wai Qi *in vitro* on cultures of human lymphocytes and human K 562 leukemia cells. Significantly, in both experiments, the effect of Wai Qi was to preserve the lymphocytes and to destroy the leukemia cells.

Other work, published in *Nature*, showed the possibility of increasing the cAMP of peripheral blood *in vitro* with Wai Qi (5).

Effects of Wai Qi on Living Creatures

Multiple experiments were carried out in China:

- on animals inoculated with cancer cells to develop a malignant process and to attempt to inhibit this malignant process with Wai Qi;
- on human cancer patients (with no control group) to attempt to arrest the development of the malignant process; and
- in healthy human subjects, to measure evidence of a physiological response to the Wai Qi stimulation.

Yang Jin Hong of Canton (6) experimented with the application of Wai Qi to healthy individuals and observed an increase of the reaction to the stimulation by PHA, and a 72 percent increase of GI value.

Jin Guan of Hangzhou (7) argues for the existence of a "Y-ray," a physical entity of biological origin and comparable to the X-ray in its destructiveness to cancer cells. With this "Y-ray," the opportunity also exists to explore the tumor, its placement and its volume.

Feng Li Da, Chairman of the Scientific Committee of the Second International Symposium of Qi Gong, inaugurated the conference on September 10th, 1989 at Xian with research results from the Center of Immunological Research of Beijing (8). The experimental results on sheep blood revealed no significant net increase in phagocytic power of peritoneal macrophages. However, the activity of the acid phosphatase of macrophages was significantly elevated (p 0.05). There was a stimulation of PFC response, anti-IGM antibodies, and an increase in the number of cells and serum Lysozyme. In mice, there was significant evidence of strengthened immune system functions in mice treated with Wai Qi. Li Cx published a similar study in *Nature* in 1983 on the phagocytic power of peritoneal macrophages (9).

Lin Bing Sui and six other researchers of the Department of Oncology of the Medical College of Tian Jin and the Institute of Bei Yan Qi Gong of the University of Tian Jin (10) carried out five studies in which the volume of tumors was decreased in rats: mammary adenocarcinoma and pulmonary adenocarcinoma. The tumors had been reduced in comparison with controls in various proportions: 58.13, 51, 44, 34.76 and 23.8 percent. The sensitivity to Wai Qi of the two types of tumors was clearly different, with the the sensitivity of pulmonary adenocarcinoma being clearly greater.

The Effects of Qi Gong Exercises on Immunity

In the twelve articles, different techniques of Qi Gong are studied, the best known being:

- He Huen Zhang Gong (sexual Qi Gong);
- Tai Ji Quan;
- Zhang Zhong Gong;
- Tai Ji Qi Gong;
- Zhou Tian Ming Men Gong; and
- Shao Lin Nei Jin Yi Zhi Chan Gong.

Certain authors conduct their studies in private hospitals, like Peng He Ming, who has recorded an abundant literature of his therapeutic experiences with his Zhi Neng Qi Gong. These experiences have not yet been translated from Chinese.

Da Huang Sheng, et. al. (11), presented to the International Symposium of Traditional Chinese Medicine and Pharmacology at Shanghai in 1987 the effects of Qi Gong exercises on the production of interferon. The method of Qi Gong was not detailed in this presentation.

In a group of 45 subjects suffering from chronic bronchitis or emphysema, the interferon response was measured before and after five months of Qi Gong training. Before the five months of Qi Gong exercises, interferon response in the group was present in only nine of the subjects. After five months of Qi Gong exercises, interferon response appeared in all subjects with a mean activity levels between 1.02 μ/ml to 11.36 μ/ml (p 0.01).

There was no interferon reaction found In a group of 50 cancer patients, prior to the Qi Gong exercises. After four months of Qi Gong exercises, 20 of 22 patients analyzed showed increase interferon levels with a mean value of 5.7 μ/ml.

In a third group of 70 "normal" (no chronic or life-threatening illnesses) subjects, there were no significant rises in interferon levels after six months of Qi Gong exercises when compared with a control group.

Xu Hefen, Qui Hue Qin, et. al. (12), studied immunological parameters of a group of patients performing Qi Gong activities. The patients, suffering from various cancers (cancers of the esophagus, stomach, lungs liver, rectum and breast) were compared to a control group of patients suffering from various cancers and who did not practice Qi Gong. Parameters studied in both groups included IgG-IgA-IgM, leukocyte adherence inhibition test (LAI), rosette formation (Ea), and the anaphthyl acetate test (ANAE). The level of IgG and the rosette test were significantly elevated in the group practicing Qi Gong, but IgA and IgM levels were not. The mean of the ANAE had been studied among the normal subjects. A significantly higher level of ANAE was demonstrated in this study with the Qi Gong practitioners (74.9 percent) compared to those who were not practicing (65.5 percent).

Luang Ren Zhong, Shen Taiwan, Jing Chengyan and Wang Jun Mei (13, 14, 15, 16) have found similar results in certain parameters such as those analyzed in the two articles mentioned above.

Hou Kung, et. al. (17), introduced the Qi Gong method called Zhou Tian Ming Men Gong to 80 cancer patients. Twenty-five patients were treated with anticancer chemotherapy, 25 were treated with chemotherapy and Qi Gong, and 30 were treated with Qi Gong alone.

The group that practiced Qi Gong as the only treatment showed increased numbers of erythrocytes, leukocytes and hemoglobin levels. The group treated with chemotherapy and Qi Gong also showed increased numbers of erythrocytes, platelets and hemoglobin, although leukocytes were not as high as in the Qi Gong-only treatment group. The group treated only with chemotherapy showed a very significant decrease in red and white blood cells, hemoglobin and platelets.

Huang Yan of Sun Yat Sen University of Medical Sciences (18) studied the augmentation of anti-infectious capacity of Qi Gong or Tai Ji Quan in healthy students. After a month of Qi Gong, significant increases were observed in salivary lysozyme and the complement C3 levels. In the Tai Ji Quan group, IgG-IgA-IgM and salivary lysozyme were increased to an equally significant degree.

Jiang Li Rui and Tao Chin (19) worked in the same manner with a group of healthy students at the Medical College of Weifang. The method of Qi Gong used was Shao Lin Nei Jin Yi Zhi Chan Gong. Blood was taken before and after these exercise groups. The investigation measured cortisol and its receptors.The levels of cortisol decreased from 7àà - 35.78 ng/dl to 1-8.85 ng/dl. At the same time, the glucocorticoid receptors increased from 3272-5152/cell to 4093-5855/cell.

Yue Qian , et. al. (20), reported a significant increase of electrophoresis of lymphocytes in healthy students after a year of practicing Shao Lin Nia Jin Ye Zhan Qi Gong.

Zhang Yong (21) of the People's Hospital of Sonzi Country, using a "spontaneous" method of Qi Gong with 16 volunteers, similar variations to the studies cited above were found for immune protein levels.

Jang Ja Ming (22) of Jiang Su made similar observations in a study with 25 students.

Conclusions

The influence of energy emitted by practitioners of Qi Gong *in vitro* and in living beings appears to have a favorable influence on immunity. The majority of factors tested take into consideration immune activity parameters such as the leucocyte count, splenic cells, lymphocyte activity, secretion of immunoglobulins and interferon activity. These parameters are positively influenced to a significant degree in the majority of experiments performed by these authors.

These studies suggest the need for further in-depth investigation in elucidating the mechanism of action of Qi Gong. These studies also suggest practical applications to preventive medicine through regulating the psychoimmunological reactions in healthy persons and also to primary and adjunctive treatments for immune deficient patients.

Notes

1) Ye Ming, et.al., "*In Vitro* Effect of 'External Qi' on Human Peripheral Blood Lymphocytes," International Conference on TCM and Pharmacology, Shanghai,. 1987: 1012-3.

2) Bi Aihua, Fang Jianming, Jiao Qinan, Liu Xiaoguang, "The Effect of the Outgoing Qi on the Expression of Surface Antigens on Human Peripheral Lymphocytes," 2nd International Conference on Qi Gong, Xian, 10-15 September 1989: 29.

3) Hu Zonglian, Chen Huiying, Jiang Shufang, "Observation of Chinese Qi Gong (Lu Ho Kuen Outer Qi) on Inducers of Terminal Granulocyte Differentiation of the Human Promyelocytic Leukemic Cell Line, Hl-Sa," 2nd International Conference on Qi Gong, Xian, 10-15 September 1989: 95.

4) Guan Hao Ben, Yang Jinhong, "Effect of External Qi by Qi Gong on Human Lymphocyte and Tumor Cells *In Vitro*," 2nd International Conference on Qi Gong, Xian, 10-15 September 1989: 98.

5) Luo, S., Huang, R.S., Wang, X.T., Chai, S.A., Yang, C.Y., "Preliminaary Experimental Observations of the Effect of Qi Gong Wai Qi on the Plasma cAMP, *Nature*, 1982.

6) Yang, Jin Hong, et. al., "Research on Action of Extra-Organismal Qi on reacti, *Acta Medica Sinica*, 1988: 3(6), 11.

7) Jin Guan, "Rayons Y et Traitement du Cancer par Qi Gong," *Science et Qi Gong*, September 1984: 8-9.

8) Feng Lid, Wang Yunsheng, Chen Shuying, Chen Haixing, "The Effect on the Immune Functions in Mice by Qi Gong 'Wai Qi,'" 2nd International Conference on Qi Gong, Xian, 10-15 September 1989: 1.

9) Li Cx, Jing I., Zhao K., "Study of Qi Gong Wai Qi-i on Phagocytic Function of Mouse Peritoneal Macrophages," *Nature*, 1983.

10) Lin Bingsui, Dou Guirong, Cui Zhenhuan, Yun Shulan, "Studies of the Mice Tumors Treated by Qi Gong Wai Qi," 2nd International Conference on Qi Gong, Xian, 10-15 September 1989: 72.

11) Da Hua Seng, et.al., "Experimental Study on Induction of Interferons in Human Body by Qi Gong," International Conference on TCM and Pharmacology, Shanghai, 1987: 1018-9.

12) Xu Hefen, et. al., "Preliminary Study on Qi Gong and Immunity," International Conference on TCM and Pharmacology, Shanghai, 1987: 993-5 and 99 of the abstracts.

13) Luan Ren Zhoung, "Observation of the Changes of Egg White IgM by Qi Gong," *Qi Gong and Sport*, 1989: 5-9.

14) Shen Zaiwen, et.al., "Influence de la Pratique des Exercices de Respiration Profonde," *Shanghai Journal of TCM*, 1984: 1-48.

15) Jing Chengyan, "Immunologie et Qi Gong," *Qi Gong et Science*, 1984: 6-3.

16) Wang Jun Mei, et. al., "Immunité et Qi Gong," *Qi Gong et Science*, 1984: 6-3.

17) Hou King, "Observations Expérimentales sur le Traitement des Tumeurs Malignes à l'Aide du Zou Tian Ming Men Gong," *Revue Qi Gong*, May 1986, Vol. 7: 101-2.

18) Huang Yan, "Research on the Relationship Between Immunity of the Human Body and Physical Training, Tai Ji Quan and Qi Gong," 2nd International Conference on Qi Gong, Xian, 10-15 September 1989: 36

19) Jian Lirui, Tao Chun, "Effect of Qi Gong on the Glucocorticoid Receptors of Human Peripheral Blood Lymphocytes and the Concentration of Cortisol," 2nd International Conference on Qi Gong, Xian, 10-15 September 1989: 56

20) Yue Qian, Zhao Shumei, Ma Weili, Wu Guoqing, "Study of Effect on Normal Numan Peripheral Blood Lymphocyte by Shao Lin Nia Jin Ye Zhi Zhan Qi Gong," 2nd International Conference on Qi Gong, Xian, 10-15 September 1989: 64.

21) Zhang Yong, Luo Shipin, Wu Yalin, "Preliminary Observation on Influence of Spontaneous Wuqinbxi Qi Gong on Human Immune Function," 2nd International Conference on Qi Gong, Xian, 10-15 September 1989: 101.

22) Jang Jamin, "A Brief View of Kong Jin Qi Gong's Influence on Immunologic Function," 2nd International Conference on Qi Gong, Xian, 10-15 September 1989: 131.

Chiropractic

Introduction

Health care can be divided into holistic and non-holistic approaches. Holistic methods use the body's inherent ability to heal itself as the basis for healing. Holistic health care incorporates a plan of treatment that does not introduce external substances into the body. Holistic approaches maintain that when the interference or blockage of the innate healing intelligence is removed, then the body can heal. The holistic concept is a viable and common means of restoring health. Chiropractic is a holistic discipline. It is one of a number of alternative methods used to restore health. Health care alternatives, including medicine, all aspire to benefit the health of the patient. The difference is that the medical alternative utilizes external chemicals designed to create internal change. Although there is a wide difference between holistic and medical approaches, both systems have years of positive results to confirm the validity of their methods.

Chiropractic as a discipline combines science, art and philosophy. The science of Chiropractic involves a methodological approach to vertebral misalignment and its resultant interference in the nervous system as the basis for the development of disease. The art of Chiropractic is a hands-on healing method. Each individual practitioner develops a style that expresses his or her own understandings and perceptions of the individual patient. The philosophy of Chiropractic emerges from the core belief that the innate healing ability of the body can be blocked by a spinal misalignment and that correction of the misalignment by the Chiropractic adjustment releases that innate healing intelligence so that the body can heal itself.

In 1895, Chiropractic was first applied with the first adjustment (vertebral manipulation) and healing of an individual's deafness. From this event, the entire field of Chiropractic emerged. The development of Chiropractic into the influential healing profession it has become is due to Chiropractic's acknowledgment of the body's ability to heal itself. It is the stimulation of this innate healing ability that generates internal wellness. This is the root of all holistic treatment.

Chiropractic care of people with AIDS, people who are HIV+ and others with immune dysfunction is multifaceted. Chiropractic's affect on the immune system, along with its affect on specific secondary symptomatology is notable. Recent research and case history analysis suggests that vertebral manipulation may have wide-ranging effects. From improvement in symptoms like peripheral neuropathy to stimulation of immune system components, Chiropractic encourages individual well-being. Quality of life issues, prevention of disease and symptoms, as well as generalized health maintenance, are the primary aspects of Chiropractic treatment. As a holistic health care alternative, a primary focus of Chiropractic is the maintenance of good health. The reduction of stress, education of an immunopositive lifestyle and the removal of nervous system interference are the central benefits Chiropractic offers.

What is Chiropractic?

Chiropractic literally means healing practice by hand. Chiropractic is based in the science, art and philosophy of vertebral manipulation as a dynamic and powerful healing discipline. The body, being constantly subjected to stress, accumulates stress. Where does it go? What do we do with it? How can we keep it from building up in our tissues to the point where disease results? These are the fundamental questions that Chiropractic seeks to answer.

Stress, although sometimes overgeneralized, is a real experience that creates tension, excitation or irritability for our body. Most stress can be accommodated by the body. We naturally adapt to stress. For example, if we are startled by a loud noise, we pull away instinctively from that noise. Our head may tilt to the side, we may cover our ears, or maybe our body will jolt. Some action occurs to disperse the stress. Under all normal circumstances and in an optimum functioning body, we can adapt to stress. Stress is an ongoing experience that our bodies usually can disperse day after day. But, when our adaptation mechanisms wear down or cannot adapt to great amounts of stress, the body begins to accumulate and store stress. Where the body accumulates stress is not always understood. However, the development of disease symptomatology is evidence that stress does manifest itself in the body. Infection is stress. In uncontrolled numbers, microbial populations can overwhelm the body. But, how does all of this pertain to Chiropractic? Chiropractic is a science, art and philosophy of vertebral manipulation.

It is the vertebral misalignment or subluxation that Chiropractic corrects. In Chiropractic, it is the subluxation that is the method or location representing the body's accumulation of stress. In Chiropractic, there are three fundamental methods of developing subluxations. These three "stresses" are structural, chemical and emotional. Structural stress includes postural, occupational and physical body exertions. Chemical stress encompasses those substances that are introduced into the body such as smoke, drugs, contaminants or other foreign antigens. Emotional stress is generated by the psyche and generally includes all situations that create emotional reactions.

The occurrence of the subluxation results in a change in the nervous system. This happens because the spine and the spinal cord are situated in an intimate relationship with one another. Due to ligamentous attachment and close proximity with the central nervous system, changes in the structural position of the spinal vertebrae result in alterations of nervous system transmissions. This relationship between the spinal vertebrae and the nervous system is the fundamental principle of Chiropractic. The subluxation (vertebral misalignment) is the primary result of stress accumulation in the body. The subluxation causes a number of changes to occur within the body. First, a spinal misalignment creates a change in the weight bearing mechanism of the body's system of balance. The subluxation creates a compression imbalance resulting in numerous physiological changes. Research in the field of compression physiology indicates that nerve root compression creates chemical and behavioral changes in the nerves. It is suspected that both static and dynamic, irritative compressions can result in a number of pathological conditions (Haldeman, 1980). Additional double-blind experimentation shows that patients diagnosed as having subluxation experience changes in sensory and motor function. Chiropractic treatment of these individuals resulted in enhanced nervous system function (Mazzarelli, 1985). The consequences of nerve root compression and the resulting nervous system changes are largely attributed to inflammation, edema and resultant anoxia that occurs within and proximal to the nerve root.

How Does Chiropractic Work?

Having now established what Chiropractic treats and why the condition of vertebral misalignment results, let's look at how a Chiropractor treats that misalignment. The correction of the subluxation is accomplished through the Chiropractic adjustment. Adjustment is the term used in Chiropractic to describe vertebral manipulation. This is the process of repositioning a misaligned vertebra by hand. There are a variety of techniques and individual methods of adjusting. The techniques and methods create the basis for the art of Chiropractic. Each individual practitioner is trained to select the technique or method that will best correct a specific subluxation, creating an individual experience with each patient. When beginning a Chiropractic analysis, the spine is evaluated using motion and static palpation to determine the extent and location of subluxations. Radiography is also widely used to confirm and substantiate the exact positioning of misaligned vertebra. The methods for detection of the subluxation have become more exact in recent years. Along with a system of radiograph marking and angle measurements, the introduction of new, computer-run thermography equipment has enabled Chiropractors to detect subluxations using thermal variations in intrinsic musculature and related soft tissue. These new methods for the detection of subluxation have improved the specific identification and location of misalignments.

Correction of the subluxation is a personal and individual practice. Individuality makes Chiropractic an art, because each practitioner develops a style based on their affinity to particular techniques. In addition, each person who receives Chiropractic care is unique. This adds to the creative process of hands-on healing. Within all the methods of correcting the subluxation, all Chiropractors adjust vertebral misalignments (subluxations) in order to normalize the nervous system. This normalization of the nervous system opens the communication between body tissues and allows innate healing to occur.

Different regions of the spine correlate with different areas of the body. The figure on page 125 diagrams corresponding areas on the spine and the associated complications that may develop if a subluxation is present in those areas. The exact mechanisms of nervous system control over body tissues is entirely more complicated than a simple one-on-one schematic representation. But, this serves as a starting point in developing an understanding of the holistic interconnectedness of the spine, nerves and resulting body function.

The Chiropractic adjustment restores the integrity of vertebral structure and normalizes nervous system control. Adjunctive therapy is often used to maximize the effect and longevity of misalignment correction. These adjuncts include massage, heat therapy, cryotherapy, manual traction, as well as mechanical therapy, including ultrasound and electrostimulation. Utilizing a combination of therapies modifies soft tissue involvement through relaxation. The comprehensive treatment of the spine, related musculature, soft tissue and implicated subluxation complex is the basis for Chiropractic as a healing discipline. The subluxation and nervous system interference, which is the result of accumulated stress, is a cause for the development of disease within the body. It is through the Chiropractic adjustment that the body is relieved of unhealthy interference in the nervous system, freeing the innate healing ability.

FIGURE: Spinal regions and innervation with physiologic function and complications. (Adapted from Cottingham, J. *Healing Through Touch*, 1985, p. 54)

Cervical: head, face thyroid, upper extremities. *Conditions of these areas:* headaches, metabolic disorders, arm and hand problems.

Thoracics: vital organs, heart, lungs, thymus, spleen. *Conditions of these areas:* immunological dysfunction, troubles with stomach, kidneys, lungs.

Lumbars: digestive organs, low back, reproductive organs. *Conditions of these areas:* bowels, uterus, prostate, low back

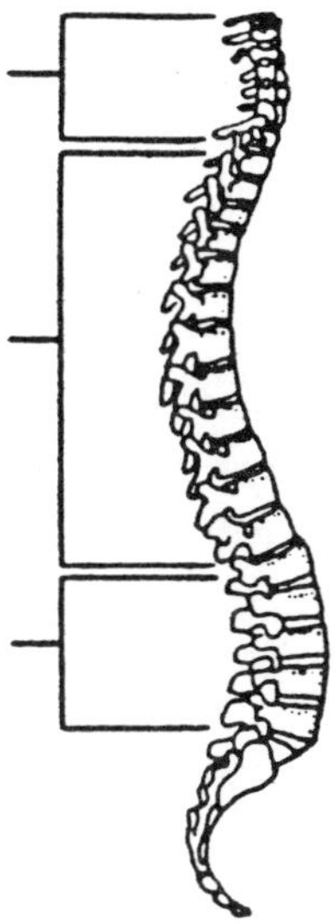

History of Chiropractic

The discovery of modern Chiropractic is attributed to D.D. Palmer in 1895. Palmer, who was a self-educated healer, acted on a supposition he had observed and he delivered the first adjustment to a deaf janitor in the building where he worked. Palmer surmised that the brain and the nervous system controlled the function and health of the body. That connection led to the theory that interference in the condition of the spine might result in disease. The janitor regained his hearing after the adjustment in what was considered a miracle healing. From that point, D.D. Palmer developed his theory into a philosophy of Chiropractic. In 1910, he published *The Science, Art and Philosophy of Chiropractic*, which remains today a widely used reference. Palmer wrote that his approach to health involved the spine, spinal adjusting and the reestablishment of normal nervous system function, without the use of drugs or instruments. D.D. Palmer's son, B.J., picked up where his father left off by creating a widely discussed an heard message that Chiropractic was a powerful healing method. B.J. Palmer created and developed a network of Chiropractic colleges and a radio station network that touted the benefits of Chiropractic to a large audience. It was B.J. who developed Chiropractic into the large and widely accepted profession that it is today. Through his consistent defense of the theories and principles established by his father, B.J. was able to further the scientific basis for Chiropractic.

Chiropractic colleges began educating individuals in the methods and techniques of manipulation therapy and gained in popularity. Within a short time, enrollment in these schools had grown significantly. As others began to work with the basic principles established by the Palmers, an individualized craft began to emerge. A wide variety of methods for achieving optimal results in the correction of the subluxation were tested and employed. Many of these techniques have been well researched, documented, systematized, and are being taught in Chiropractic colleges today.

Chiropractic has recently gained wider acceptance as a legitimate and effective health care alternative. Many Chiropractors act as primary health care providers and make referrals to specialists as the need arises. In 1979, the government of New Zealand appointed a commission to investigate the efficacy of Chiropractic and possible insurance reimbursement for Chiropractic patients. Their findings are viewed as extremely positive, and they have determined that Chiropractic is a valuable branch of health care. It wasn't until the late 1970s that the United States granted insurability to Chiropractic on the basis of years of subjective patient wellness and sound clinical evidence to support Chiropractic principles.

In the 1980s, the American Medical Association and affiliated organizations lost a multimillion dollar lawsuit brought about by Chiropractic professionals. This lawsuit contested the violation of anti-trust laws, and the propagation of false information leading the the detriment of the Chiropractic profession. There was an appeal by the medical profession, which also was lost. Presently, up to 35 million Americans use Chiropractic regularly, and there is a gaining acceptance and popularity worldwide. New international Chiropractic colleges have opened, and the number of Chiropractors in Europe, Asia and the Middle East has significantly increased.

Presently,

> the vast majority of Chiropractic patients are treated for back, neck and shoulder complaints, as well as minor headaches. Some 10 percent seek help for organic diseases of all sorts. (Purvis, A., *Time*, September 23, 1991, p. 61)

Chiropractic care, D.D. Palmer asserted, is for the treatment of all disease, including organic illness. Case histories reveal improvement in a variety of organic conditions including asthma, allergies, digestive disorders and some gynecological irregularities. Over time, there has been an attempt to reduce and limit Chiropractic to spinal conditions. This compartmentalization of Chiropractic into a simple remedy for spinal ailments is in part dues to the years of medical oppression, along with self-assumed restrictions in scope of practice.

> It is to the public detriment that too large a segment of Chiropractic profession is abdicating the role of the Chiropractic physician for the less demanding musculoskeletal specialization. (Homewood, 1981, p. 20)

Chiropractic and Immunity

Up to this point, we have examined the principles, origins and legitimacy of Chiropractic as a healing method. Now we need to take those principles and apply them to the topic at hand, namely AIDS, HIV infection, and the integrity of the immune system. Nathaniel Altman notes that in *Psychoimmunity and the Healing Process*, edited by Jason Serinus, Chiropractic alignment of the body, specifically to alleviate stress and tensions placed on the medulla oblongata and the coccyx, is important in cases of

AIDS and other immune dysfunction. Chiropractic adjustments open up neurological pathways to help restore the proper functioning of the nervous and endocrine systems of the body. (Altman, N. p. 18)

The results of Chiropractic adjusting on these two areas affects large numbers of nerves, either as part of the spinal cord that merges with the lower brain stem (medulla oblongata) or the ganglionic collection of nerves found near the coccyx. The opening up of neurologic pathways that Altman refers to seems to be achieved most effectively when these principal areas of the spine are adjusted. The answer to why this could be involves an understanding of the importance of the medulla oblongata and the coccygeal ganglion. Both are composed of large clusters of nerves that control involuntary functions of vital body processes. In the case of the medulla oblongata, numerous connections between areas of the brain occur. Chiropractic adjusting in these areas frees those crucial regulatory centers.

Altman goes on to say that Tom O'Connor, who was diagnosed with ARC, included Chiropractic in his health care program,. In his book, *Living with AIDS*, O'Connor spoke highly of Chiropractic. Not only did he derive great benefits from his treatments, he also stated that Chiropractic enhanced his sense of responsibility for the health of his body. He determined that a visit to a competent Chiropractor should benefit anyone, especially those whose immune systems cannot afford to be further impaired by a structural nervous dysfunction. (Altman, N. 1990, p. 19) These sources imply that Chiropractic adjustments may directly affect the immune system in a positive direction. Serinus and O'Connor also indicate that spinal misalignment and resulting nervous system interference are a hindrance to normal immune system function, since they place an abnormal stress on the body. One point worth noting is that retroviral activity is particularly increased under conditions of stress. As an example, herpes simplex virus expresses itself as a vesicular lesion more often under immunosuppressive conditions (i.e., solar exposure, fever, common cold, anxiety, drug use, profuse emotional stress). The implication of this is that HIV activity may also be increased in an environment of abnormally stressful conditions. In a holistic approach, this concept is substantial, because the grounds for illness originate with the formation of an unsuitable atmosphere for wellness.

A direct relationship between the functioning of the immune system and Chiropractic can be made. There have been several studies that support the theory that immune function is affected by the intact performance of the nervous system. Mark Mead, in his article on Chiropractic, cites research done by Ronald Pero, Ph.D., Chief of Cancer Prevention Research at New York's Preventive Medicine Institute and Professor of Medicine in Environmental Health at New York University:

> Chiropractic patients in his [Pero's] study had 200 percent greater immune competence than people who had not received Chiropractic, and 400 percent greater immune competence than people with other serious disease.

He further states that:

> Chiropractic may optimize whatever genetic abilities you have to fully resist serious disease. (Mead, M. *East West Journal*, November 1989, p. 67)

Recent and increasingly detailed experimentation has revealed that there is enhanced and significant phagocytic respiratory bursts of polymorphonuclear neutrophils in response to particulate challenging following a single thoracic manipulation. (Nansel, D., Szlazak, M., Brennan, P.C., Triano, J.T., McGregor, M., Kokjohn, K., Kaltinger, C.J., Lohr, G.E, *JMPT*, September 1993, February 1992, January 1992) These studies present evidence that vertebral manipulation does have an effect on the immune system. They also show that this effect is positive, and that if effects can be achieved on the neutrophilic cells of the immune system, then the potential for effects on the lymphocytes is also possible and probable.

Chiropractic may also affect the immune system in an indirect manner. As mentioned before, Chiropractic care assists in the development of an immunopositive lifestyle. Additionally, Chiropractic adjusting may help to strengthen the immune system by normalizing and reinforcing the normal function of other body systems. Some of the most recent research on HIV infection indicates that internal mechanisms may in fact be assisting in the control of HIV infection. For example, vasoactive intestinal peptide (VIP), plays a multifunctional role on both the peripheral and central nervous system. VIP may in fact counteract HIV-induced neuronal cell death. (Chelbi-Alix, M..K., January 1994) VIP as an intestinal protein is manufactured under the guidance of internal regulatory systems within the body. It is the nervous system that governs these regulatory processes by providing feedback, information and communication between the brain and the involved body tissues. The response and function of various organs, including digestive functions, is affected by vertebral subluxation. (Homewood, 1981) It may be broadly assumptive to say that Chiropractic can effect the production of an internal substance that may help in counteracting the effects of HIV. Yet, this is a rationale that develops from the holistic understanding that the body has an internal method of handling disease.

Homewood goes on to reference several other researchers who have shown marked results in their investigations. Most notably, A.N. Gordienko, et.al, showed that the nervous system was essential for the reception of the stimulus of the antigen, and that the autonomic division and the Vagus nerve give evidence of being the controlling system for immunity. (Homewood, 1981) Homewood also quotes Kuntz in stating that:

> The data set forth regarding the autonomic nervous influences in the distribution of leukocytes and the permeability of the vascular endothelium strongly suggests that immunity and bodily resistance, in a large measure, are determined by the functional condition of the autonomic nervous system. (Homewood, 1981, p. 295)

In light of this evidence, it is relevant to conclude that the immune system is in part regulated by the nervous system. The fact that the nervous system is affected by the presence of the vertebral misalignment has already been discussed. We can then infer that the correction of the vertebral misalignment by the Chiropractic adjustment can help and assist in the enhancement of the immune system, either directly or through the normalization of other bodily systems.

Chiropractic and the PWA

At this point in the AIDS epidemic, it is becoming increasingly clear that PWAs are seeking procedures other than traditional drugs and medical approaches to assist them with their health. The reason for this may simply be that while medical research is looking for the "answer" to this crisis, many people are still dying. It becomes apparent that the PWA is taking into account all methods of treatment that may assist or enhance the ability to be healthy. (Kessler, W.J., Blanc, P., Greenblatt, H.R., *UCSF*, 1990; Hand, R., *NEJM*, 1989,; Cassileth, B.R., Lusk, E.J., Bodenheimer, B.M., *AIM*, 1984)

Chiropractic is one of a number of choices that are available to the person seeking holistic health care. The body's ability to function, its internal wellness, is generated by the liberation of the innate healing ability. Unlocking this door through whatever method is "our" answer to assist in the prevention of an unhealthy state. Clinical experiences have led AIDS health care professionals to conclude that PWAs often want and sometimes demand education in the most effective ways to assist them with their general health as well as how to best help themselves with this infection. Chiropractors and other alternative professionals often recommend exercise, nutrition, rest, attitude, education, personal habits, along with passive assistance. Passive assistance is care that an individual might receive from someone else, such as Chiropractic, acupuncture, massage, etc.

The immunopositive lifestyle is something a PWA can develop in all those hours when they are not visiting a Chiropractor, acupuncturist, medical doctor or the myriad of other health specialists that they must utilize in order to stay ahead of the illness.

Leading the immunopositive lifestyle requires ongoing, healthy intentions and all the positive feedback that it can create. Along with Chiropractic adjustment, which is the core of Chiropractic, this encouragement and guidance is an integral part of many Chiropractor's health care objectives.

We have examined the potential effects of the Chiropractic adjustment on the immune system. There are other effects that Chiropractic can have on secondary symptomatology seen in AIDS, specifically peripheral neuropathy. Of the cases of AIDS and HIV infection that Chiropractors work with, up to 80 percent of these patients report some degree of peripheral neuropathy (i.e., numbness, tingling and/or burning in either or both of the extremities). The direct correlation between the Chiropractic adjustment and associated soft tissue therapy significantly decreases these symptoms and results in a rapid change in other symptoms. Much of this change is due to the specific cervical or lumbar manipulation therapy and distal to proximal massage of soft tissue to promote lymphatic drainage and the redistribution of tissue toxins for facilitated removal by the circulatory and lymphatic systems. Follow-up visits reveal that these changes are present for varying amounts of time, usually with positive effects remaining for up to 4-5 days. It is important to note that the redevelopment of symptoms does occur in most patients. This is probably due to the increase in toxicity within the extremities themselves, while continued treatment provides relief.

The extent of Chiropractic's benefit to the PWA is challenging to assess. Due to difficulties in developing control situations, the positive effects of the Chiropractic adjustment and soft tissue manipulation are limited. There is, however, evidence suggesting that a positive relationship does exist. With ongoing treatment and further clinical work, Chiropractic care is assisting PWAs with their health. Continued research, observation and insights will unfold the full potential of Chiropractic as a powerful healing alternative for HIV infection.

Conclusion

Chiropractic, like other alternative health care, is in the infancy of its development as a treatment for AIDS. Compared with traditional medical research, a very small amount of time and money have been invested in the research of holistic alternatives to AIDS. While the medical community searches for an external cure, Chiropractic continues to heal from within. This idea, which is the root of all holistic health, is firmly planted in the philosophy of Chiropractic. The Chiropractic method of achieving this internal wellness comes from balancing the nervous system using the Chiropractic adjustment. By balancing the nervous system, a clearer communication link is established between body tissues. This unobstructed communication then enables the body to perform its numerous functions unencumbered. The immune system, being one of these functions, is given the opportunity to act with competence.

Chiropractic has shown its ability to enhance immune system function directly and indirectly. Directly, it acts on areas of the nervous system that regulate the production and effect of immunological components. Indirectly, it effects other internal systems that have a direct effect on the immune system. On both levels, Chiropractic is engaging the body in producing an optimal healing environment.

Chiropractic treatment involves a comprehensive approach to individual wellness and assists the PWA in a number of ways. Through an evaluation of healthy lifestyle options, as well as bodywork designed to reinforce and strengthen the immune system, Chiropractic administers a health care option that is in the forefront of holistic care for HIV infection.

Bibliography

1) Kessler, W.j., Blanc, P., Greenblatt, H.R., "The Use of Medicinal Herbs Among AIDS Clinic Patients." Robert Wood Johnson Clinical Scholars Program and Department of Medicine, University of California, San Francisco, CA, International Conference on AIDS 1990, June 20, 23:6(3): 210.

2) Nansel, D., Szlazak, M. , "Enhanced Phagocytic Cell Respiratory Burst Induced by Spinal Manipulation." *Journal of Manipulative Physiologic Therapeutics*, September 1993, 16(7): 505-7.

3) Brennan, P.C., Triano, J.T., McGregor, M., KokJohn, K., "Significant Difference in the Respiratory Burt of Polymorphonuclear Neutrophils in Response to Particulate Challenge Following a Single Thoracic Manipulation." *Journal of Manipulative Physiologic Therapeutics*, February 1992, 15(2): 83-9.

4) Brennan, P.C., Kokjohn, K., Kaltinger, C.J., Lohr, G.E., "Respiratory Burst of Polymorphonuclear Neutrophils and Monocytes from Adults." *Journal of Manipulative Physiologic Therapeutics*, January 1992, 15(5): 334-5.

5) Chelbi-Alix, M.K., Bronard, A., Boissard, C., Pelapat, D., "Induction by Vasoactive Intestinal Peptide of Interferon Alpha/Beta Syntheses in Glial Cells But Not Neurons." Institute National de lal Sante et de la Recherche Medicale, Paris, France, *Journal Cell Physiology*, January 1994, 158(1): 47-54.

6) Hand, R., M.D., "Alternative Therapies Used by Patients with AIDS." *New England Journal of Medicine*, March 1989, 320(10): 672-673.

7) Cassileth, B.R., Lusk, E.J., Stroube, T.B., Bodenheimer, B.M., "Contemporary Unorthodox Treatments in Cancer Medicine: A Study of Patients, Treatments and Practitioners." *Annals of Internal Medicine*, 1984, 101: 105-12.

8) Purvis, A., "Is There a Method to Manipulation?" *Time*, September 1991, 23: 60-61.

9) Mead, M.N., "Chiropractic." *East West Journal*, November 1989:64-84.

10) Altman, N., *Chiropractic Health Care*. Los Angeles: 1990, Tarcher Publishers, 18-19.

11) Serinus, J., Ed., *Pychoimmunity and the Healing Process*. Berkeley, California: 1986, Celestial Arts.

12) Bricklin, M., *Natural Healing*. Emmaus, Pennsylvania: 1983, Rodale Press.

13) Haldeman, S., *Modern Developments in the Principals and Practice of Chiropractic*. Norwalk, Connecticut: 1980, Appleton-Century-Crofts.

14) Mazzarelli, J., Ed., *Chiropractic Interprofessional Research*. Torino, Italy: 1982, Edizioni Minerva Medica.

15) Cottingham, J., *Healing Through Touch*. Boulder, Colorado: 1985, Rolf Institute.

16) Homewood, A.E., *The Neurodynamics of Vertebral Subluxation*, 3rd Edition. St. Petersburg, Florida: 1981, Valkyrie Press, Inc.

The Role of Chiropractic

Introduction

Chiropractic was developed over 100 years ago by D.D. Palmer in Davenport, Iowa. The word, Chiropractic, is derived from the Greek "chiro praktis," meaning "the practice of the hands." it is a hands-on system of manipulation, in which the body's own natural energy is released and allowed to come through into a full expression of healing itself. Manipulation with hands has been practiced for over 2,000 years in the East. Although manipulation is not a new idea in the Eastern world, it was new to the Western world 100 years ago. It was an innovative breakthrough, which combined an Eastern approach to a Western science in a practical form. Palmer envisioned Chiropractic to be the philosophy, science and art of healing.

The philosophy states that there is a universal energy or life force that surrounds us, from which everything imaginable derives its essential being. Consider the smallest atomic particle in space to the largest mountain on earth or the deepest depths of the sea. Universal energy is boundless, connecting everything that vibrates with the same life force. It is this energy that drives the universe from order to chaos and back again.

In quantum physics, we are in a constant cyclical state of change. As soon as we identify the directional spin of an atom in space, its speed has altered and we can no longer detect it in the same location. Such is the changing nature of universal energy that we are just now beginning to tap into scientifically, with the advent of quantum physics in the Western world.

We know that matter is neither created nor destroyed. It is all part of the constant changing whole. For hundreds and thousands of years, cultures have spoken of cosmic energy and the forces of nature over which we as humans have no control. Chinese Taoism created the concept of the unifying force, "the way" or path which has no name but is all paths in one. The Taoists believed in the oneness between this earthly life plane and the hereafter as part of the same energy. In meditation, the Taoists practice the "micro cosmic orbit," to moved the internal breath/energy through the body, much as the energy is moved through the universe. This energy is called Qi or Chi.

In India, we find a similar belief system of a cosmic or universal energy. Both Ayurvedic and Hindu systems practice what is called the "cosmic breath" in meditation as well as the cosmic sound or "mantra." The breath and sound are used to unify the field of internal energy with the cosmic energy of the universe. This form of mantra meditation enables people to harmonize on a similar frequency with the universal "atomic" energy.

Chiropractic describes a similar cosmic, internal

energy or Chi and calls it "innate energy." Innate energy is the force within all beings that has its own natural rhythm and flow. It balances the state of homeostasis that is necessary for the body to function. it is the vital life force that links body, mind and spirit. We realize that we are not merely mental beings, emotional beings, physical or chemical beings, but rather, a composite of all of the above, which is governed by a breath of life. Palmer hypothesized that when this innate energy was in a balanced state, the body was in a state of health. However, when the innate energy was blocked, the body experienced a state of "dis-ease." In pathology, the disease is a state of complete confusion in which the body has lost control of its ability to contain pathogens, fight off infection or curtail the growth of abnormal cells.

Disease implies a sub-clinical state of imbalance. It is a disharmony within. The body is functioning below its optimal state but not quite in a state of pathology. Sub-clinical signs are not usually detectable by clinical tests., i.e., blood tests, X-rays, etc.. They are identifiable by patient symptomology that represent the initial stages and onset of imminent pathology. Disease of the organism can also be present when actual pathology exists. In this state, the aim is still to bring the body back into alignment. The goal is to remove any mechanical obstructions that could prevent the body from utilizing its full healing potential.

The Science of Chiropractic

In the science of Chiropractic the most crucial areas, the conveyer belts of this innate energy, are the nervous and the endocrine systems. The nervous system receives thousands of bits of information from different sensory organs and makes a determination as to what the appropriate response will be.

There are two basic divisions to the nervous system: the sensory and motor divisions.

The sensory division includes sensory receptors such as visual, auditory and tactile receptors. The information enters the nervous system through these receptors, through the skin or deep structures of the body and is transmitted through the spinal nerves to the spinal chord at all levels before reaching the brain. Sensory experience can be stored in the memory to be used to determine the body's reaction at a later date, or it can cause an immediate reaction.

The second division, known for its control of bodily activities, is the motor division. It controls the effects or motor functions of the body by contraction of skeletal muscle throughout the body and contraction of smooth muscle in the internal organs. The secretion of exocrine and endocrine glands is controlled by this motor division.

The skeletal muscles can be controlled from many different levels of the central nervous system, including the spinal cord, the reticular substance of the medulla, pons and mesencephalon, the basal ganglia, the cerebellum and the motor cortex.

A parallel system of the skeletal effector system is called the autonomic nervous system (ANS), which is comprised of the sympathetic and parasympathetic nervous systems. It is activated primarily by centers located in the spinal chord, brain stem, hypothalamus and some portions of the cerebral cortex. This system operates through visceral reflexes. Sensory signals from parts of the body transmit information to these centers and these centers relay the appropriate reflex response back to the visceral organs to control their activities. This system also governs functions such as gastrointestinal motility, urinary output, secretions, sweating, body temperature, endorphin release and many other functions, most of which are involuntary.

The sympathetic nerve pathways originate in different segments of the spinal cord (from thoracic-1 to lumbar-2) and pass out of a spinal nerve. The level of the segment from which it arises is not necessarily the same pat of the body that will be affected. The parasympathetic nervous system leaves the central nervous system through several of the cranial nerves, the first, second, third and fourth sacral nerves. Both the sympathetic and parasympathetic nervous systems can have either an excitatory or inhibitory effect on organs. For example, the sympathetic system will dilate pupils and lung bronchi while inhibiting gallbladder and bile ducts and constricting abdominal blood vessels. The parasympathetic system will contract pupils and constrict lung bronchi while exciting gallbladder, bile ducts and bladder.

There are three major levels of the nervous system:

1) the spinal cord,

2) the lower brain level, and

3) the higher brain.

In response to a sensory signal, almost all spinal cord motor responses will occur spontaneously. These patterns are called reflexes. There is a muscle stretch reflex, which will react to a sensory nerve fiber within the muscle to prevent overstretching, the muscle spindle will respond by contracting to prevent further damage. There also is a protective withdrawal reflex, which withdraws withdraws the body part from any object that is causing pain. (3)

The lower brain level is concerned mostly with what we would call the subconscious activities. It is located in the medulla, pons, mesencephalon, hypothalamus, thalamus, cerebellum and basal ganglia. It governs functions of arterial pressure and respiration, anger, excitement, sexual activities, feeding reflexes, reaction to pleasure and pain as well as the coordination of turning movements.

The higher brain (cortical level) is a vast storehouse of information. Many the patterns of motor responses and most of our past memories are stored here. About three quarters of all neuronal cell bodies are located in the cerebral cortex. In this area of the brain, we see the more developed, abstract process of thought. The brain is the master controller of the millions of electrical nerve cells that both transmit and receive messages.

Through a very intricate system of chemical and electrical charges, neurons travel along pathways and are able to relay messages that can trigger various responses. A message can originate in the brain as a conscious thought to lift the leg, or it can originate in the arm as an itching, which signals the brain that the skin needs to be scratched. Neurological pathways carry signals from the brain to the spinal cord and exit out through spinal nerves to affect muscle, tendons, fascia, organs, tissues, etc. This can effect a motor response where the muscle is governed, voluntarily or involuntarily, to contract.

The Art of Chiropractic

The art of Chiropractic is is less precisely definable. It is the beauty of the adjustment, which is delivered with the correct amount of pressure in the exact area of the body that requires it. This is that part of being known instinctively by the Chiropractic doctor after years of training and practical application. It is the exact location of pain and the correct procedure to alleviate that pain. The art of healing is more than the art of physical manipulation. It is the instinctive technique of touching, from the soft touch of palpation to the deep applied acupressure, to the more osseous, forceful thrust. Each technique is an art form in its own right.

Applied kinesiology is the study of muscles in motion and its application to their functional testing. Applied kinesiology gives a wide range of information about the integrity of not only musculo-skeletal strength but also its relationship to the peripheral and central nervous system. Additionally, it provides information regarding the association between organ function and neuro-musculo-skeletal function.

Sacro-occipital technique is an adjustment that uses blocks under the lumbar-sacrum-pelvic region to "re-pattern" the neurological message received from the sacral nerves through the soft tissue and meninges of the spinal cord to the occipital nerves of the cranium. This technique can be effective for alleviating muscle and joint pain, headaches, visual disturbances and intestinal disturbances.

Osseous adjustment is the Chiropractic technique that is most familiar to people who have received adjustments. It applies a necessary amount of pressure directly over a vertebra to deliver a thrust in a particular direction. This manipulation increases mobility of a joint or decreases inflammation, which may arise in soft tissue as a result of misaligned or subluxated vertebrae. A subluxation is defined as a mild rotation of the vertebra, usually followed by an irritation of the corresponding nerve root. The irritation of the nerve root can be followed by an inflammation of soft tissue, initiation of pain fibers being triggered, and corresponding muscle spasms and/or myofascitis. Chemically, there appears to be a release of endorphins in the skin. This chemical release often results in a feeling of well-being.

There are numerous Chiropractic techniques, using both force and non-force for adjusting or realigning the vertebra. Additionally, there are various soft tissue methods used for stretching and strengthening muscle fibers. Other methods include are used to induce deep relaxation and alpha brain-wave states. These methods involve the administering of micro-currents of electrical stimulation on ear points,

Utilization of adjunctive therapies such as moist hot and cold packs, ultrasound and electrical muscle stimulation are also included in Chiropractic care.

Treatment of HIV Infection and AIDS

In the treatment of HIV infection and AIDS, we know that there is not one answer, one drug, one cure. The effective method of treatment is to approach the person as a multi-faceted, whole being. The complexity of that statement can be bewildering, because no one really has a clue as to what makes up all of the parts of any human being. In their diligence and dedication to find answers, health care professionals can be most effective when they remember the physician's oath to "first, do no harm." That means treating everyone as human beings, as mothers, fathers, brothers and sisters, treating people as they would want to be treated themselves.

Chiropractic is a drug-free, hands-on treatment that works with the realigning or the tuning up of the body's own natural life force. Chiropractic diagnoses particular imbalances within the neuro-musculo-skeletal structure of the body and then, through varied Chiropractic techniques, fixes those imbalances. These techniques or adjustments alleviate pain and correct imbalances through a laying on of hands. Laying on hands is more than jargon. It is the actual transference of energy, from the Chiropractor to the patient. It is this person-to-person relationship which brings about the transition from a state of unwellness to a state of wellness.

If HIV infection is the unknown state of being seropositive and symptom free, then AIDS is the resulting state of chronic unwellness. In both conditions, imbalances exist. Some imbalances are hidden deep within the body and some are visible. However, the treatment approach for both conditions essentially is the same. First, identify and locate obvious and easily diagnosed problems. Second, support and continue supporting the body's own natural defense system with all available resources. This should be done in the context of the whole person. The mind, body and spirit are inseparable from that whole person.

Homeopathy

Introduction

Homeopathy is based on the "law of similars" or "like cures like." In homeopathic medicine, the practitioner (homeopath) determines the substances that cause similar symptoms to those found in a sick patient. Once the homeopath has determined the appropriate medicine, it is prescribed in microdoses (or minute doses). These doses are thought to stimulate the immune system so that the body's own defense mechanism can create antibodies. In classical homeopathy, a homeopath diagnoses a person's physical and psychological symptoms and prescribes a single medicine in microdoses. One unconventional approach to homeopathy is based on a combination of medicines. In this instance, a homeopath might combine three to eight types of medicines. (1) The concept that like cures like is not foreign to conventional medicine. Indeed, many vaccines are based on this principle. Certain vaccines protect against disease because they contain minute amounts of a virus that in greater quantities would produce severe illness. An example of minute doses in conventional medicine is the use of the homeopathic approach in the treatment of allergies, in which allergens are used to induce an antibody response. (2)

Historical Overview of Homeopathy in the United States

The Law of Similars, *Similia Similbus Curentur*, or "let likes be cured by likes," was first postulated by Hippocrates. However, it was not developed into a unique scientific system of medicine until 1796, when a German physician, Samuel Hahneman, established homeopathy. (3) Homeopathy was introduced into the United States by Hans Gram, a Dutch homeopath, in 1825. The initial practitioners of homeopathy in the United States were medical school graduates from Harvard, Dartmouth and other prestigious schools. (4) Homeopathy became so popular that the first national medical society was established, the American Institute of Homeopathy (AIH) in 1844. The American Medical Association was established in 1846.

Homeopathy became popular because it was successful in treating the various epidemic diseases that occurred in Europe and America in the 1800s. (5) Homeopathy was very effective in controlling cholera and yellow fever outbreaks. Statistics indicate that death rates from these epidemics in homeopathic hospitals were often half to as little as one-eighth of those in orthodox medical hospitals. (6) In Cincinnati, homeopathic doctors were so successful in treating people during the cholera epidemic of 1848, that only 3 percent of the 1,116 homeopathic patients died, while between 48 and 60 percent of those under orthodox medical treatment died.

By 1900, homeopathy was a very well established

and accepted modality of treatment. There were 22 homeopathic medical schools, ove 100 homeopathic hospitals and more than 1,000 homeopathic pharmacies in the United States. Unlike the orthodox medical establishment, homeopathic practitioners were open to the idea of allowing women to practice homeopathy. Homeopathic medical schools began accepting women in 1871. The AMA did not invite women into its organization until 1915. (9) Homeopathy not only had grass roots support but it attracted support from many of the most respected members of society, including Henry Wadsorth Longfellow, Nathaniel Hawthorne, Harriet Beecher Stowe, Daniel Webster, William Seward and Louisa May Alcott. (10)

A renowned homeopath, Dana Ullman, has recounted the well-documented history of opposition to homeopathy from the ranks of orthodox medical practitioners. Initially, the animosity arose because of criticism by homeopaths of conventional medicine. Homeopathy offered an integrated, systematic and coherent basis for its therapeutic practice. But, because of opposition by medical practitioners and also because of economics, homeopathy declined. In an AMA meeting in 1903, one of the more respected orthodox physicians stated, "We must admit that we never fought the homeopaths on matters of principles; we fought them because they came into the community and got the business." (11) The resistance to homeopathy within the ranks of the AMA became so visceral that many physicians who were homeopaths were excluded from the local medical societies that controlled licensure. In 1855, the AMA established a "consultation clause" within their code of ethics, which asserted that orthodox physicians would lose their membership in AMA if they even consulted with a homeopath or any other "nonregular" practitioner.

Due to the AMA's stance, there was a decline in homeopathy in the United States. The decline of homeopathic schools can be traced to concerted efforts by the AMA to invalidate homeopathic medical schools and prevent homeopathic graduates from being able to take qualifying boards for licensure. In 1910, the Flexner report conducted by the Carnegie Foundation in cooperation with members of the AMA rated all the medical schools in the country and gave homeopathic schools low ratings. (13) As a result of that report, only graduates of homeopathic schools with the highest marks were allowed to take medical licensing boards. By 1923, there were only two homeopathic schools left in the country. (14) Furthermore, another factor contributing to homeopathy's decline was that orthodox medical practitioners began incorporating certain homeopathic principles in their practice. Finally, orthodox medicine was more financially profitable than homeopathy, which is a more time-consuming practice, due to the nature of homeopathic treatment.

Homeopathy in Europe

There is a greater acceptance of homeopathy in Europe. In a survey of recently graduated British physicians, conducted by the *British Medical Journal*, 80 percent expressed an interest in being trained in either homeopathy or acupuncture. There are a number of physicians in England who also refer their patients of homeopathic physicians. In France, a recent survey revealed that 11,000 physicians utilize homeopathic medicines. Around 20,000 French pharmacies sell homeopathic medicines. This is because homeopathy is taught in all French schools of pharmacy and approximately 1,000 French physicians specialize in homeopathy. In that same survey, it was estimated that approximately 25 percent of the French public has tried or is presently using homeopathic medicines. Homeopathy also is popular in many countries in Latin America and Asia. (15)

Mechanism of Homeopathy

There is no scientific explanation of how homeopathic medicines function in the body. However, "it should be acknowledged that pharmacologists today do not understand why most conventional drugs work, despite all the money spent on research." (16) The pharmaceutical process of manufacturing homeopathic medicine is known as *potentization.* Potentization is a procedure of repeated (serial) dilutions of a medicinal substance in 99 parts of distilled water or ethyl alcohol. One part of the first dilution is further diluted with 99 parts of distilled water or ethyl alcohol, and then shaken. This dilution process can occur numerous times, hence the appellation, serial dilution. (17) Homeopaths admit that after numerous dilutions, there might not even be a molecule of the medicinal substance left in the water or alcohol solvent. It is therefore difficult to understand the process of pharmacologicl effect if there is no medicinal substance except alcohol or water in the solution. (18) Homeopaths believe that even though there might not be any medicinal substance in the homeopathic preparation, the solution contains a pattern or energy of the medicinal substance, which carries with it curative effects.

Homeopathic medicines are criticized for their lack of uniformity in composition because of the processes whereby they are produced. Dr. Kleijnen and Dr. Reit, two Dutch physicians from the Department of Epidemiology and Health Care Research at the

University of Limburg note that the process of producing homeopathic preparations differs greatly among manufacturers. (19) However, homeopaths have documented the effects of drugs, which are compiled into *materia medicas* (medical encyclopedias) and other books that list symptoms with substances found to cause or cure a wide variety of ailments. The *Homeopathic Pharmacopoeia of the United States* is a standard reference text that details the sources, composition and preparation of homeopathic medicines that are prescribed according to the standard Homeopathic Law of Similars. (21) Homeopaths do indeed utilize a very organized and systematic approach in the preparation of medicines and the prescription of these medicines to effect specific illnesses and conditions of the human body.

Homeopathy in the Treatment of HIV/AIDS

Controlled research conducted on the efficacy of homeopathy in the treatment of HIV/AIDS has been scarce. (22) Past research has demonstrated that homeopathy has been effective in treating rheumatoid arthritis and other immune disorders. There is a general consensus, according to Dana Ullman, that homeopathy has little to offer an individual with end-stage AIDS. As of mid-1987, there were at least 250 people with AIDS under homeopathic care. However, there has been no evaluation on the condition of these people. (23

The scarcity of research data on homeopathic medicines and their possible therapeutic effects on HIV/AIDS is a gap that Leanna Standish, Director of Research at Bastyr University in Seattle, is seeking to rectify. Dr. Standish believes that there is an urgent need for publishing research on homeopathic remedies in the treatment of HIV/AIDS patients and is attempting to collect data from studies that other researchers are pursuing.

A final report of a very successful HIV/AIDS pilot study has caught the interest of Dr. Standish. This study utilized a highly effective, natural and non-toxic new modality that combines the best of Western technology with centuries-old healing techniques of the East: herbalism, homeopathy, acupuncture and micro-pulsed electronic stimulation. It already has qualified for patent protection in the United States, Europe and many other countries.

Of the 29 different clinical study reports that she has reviewed, Dr. Standish reports that this modality showed the most significant improvement in generally accepted HIV/AIDS markers. For example, there was a marked improvement in T4 cell levels, with 85.6% of the patients having increased or stable counts during the first 10 months of the study. This pattern of improvement continued during the following 22-29 months. Additionally, almost every patient in the study had substantial increase in their responses to delayed-type hypersensitivity skin tests. This is virtually unheard of with current HIV/AIDS drugs.

The original pilot study of this exciting and promising new therapy was conducted in the United States with European funding. However, due to the general lack of interest in alternative medicine in this country, it has appeared that the impending follow-up study will be conducted in London.

At a time when very little positive research has been reported and with the recent shifts in attitudes in the United States toward natural medicine with endorsements of university and government organizations, treatment breakthroughs such as this could be kept at home. The investigators , who want to maintain confidentiality until final study results have been made public in a press conference in mid-July, hope to be able to identify American funding sources for the next clinical trial.

In a telephone conversation on June 29, 1994, with Dr. Leanna Standish, Director of Research at Bastyr University, she reported on a 5-year open trial that was conducted on 30 early symptomatic HIV+ patients. The patients received a combination of hydrotherapy, nutritional medicine and counseling. Half of the patients received either botanical or homeopathic remedies. The results of the trial indicate that there were symptomatic improvements and a transient rise in CD_4 counts in trial participants at 3 months. After one year, there was no progression to AIDS and no deaths among trial participants. The 5-year evaluation of the trial in 1994 indicates that among all of the trial participants there was a slowed progression of the disease and a decrease in mortality relative to epidemiological statistics for Seattle/King County. These results are promising. However, it is difficult to determine the efficacy of homeopathic treatment, as it was a part of a combination treatment. While this trial sample is too small to make definitive conclusions, it does provide the impetus for further trials being conducted on a large scale.

In a study conducted in 1987 by Lawrence E. Badgley, MD, homeopathic remedies were used on 10 self-selected patients. Single homeopathic remedies were chosen and prescribed to each patient. The method chosen to identify which remedy to prescribe was accomplished through the following procedure. The patient was placed in a supine position on an examination table and individual remedies were presented near the patient's body field while the practitioner palpated the patient's radial pulse for the vascular autonomic signal (VAS) reflex. (24) A remedy that aroused the VAS reflex was chosen for therapeutic prescription. T-cell lymphocyte profiles were obtained prior to ingestion of the remedy and various times afterwards. The follow-up was conducted for 2-9 months after treatment. In three of the patients, there was a significant improvement in T4 / T8 lymphocyte profiles and none of the patients died. Therapeutic benefits were seen in both high and low potency medicines. Improvements in T-cell lymphocyte profiles generally occurred 2-12 weeks after ingesting the medicine. This effect period of the medicine is quite often the case in homeopathic treatment. The remedy most commonly prescribed was Typhoidinum. Dr. Badgley suggests that the HIV virus might be similar to typhoid. The general order of application that was discovered in this study was Badiaga, Mercuris, Cyclosporine and Typhoidinum. (25)

Other studies are being conducted in Europe and Asia with homeopathic medicines in the treatment of HIV/AIDS. In England, Michael Strange, a homeopath, has 45 HIV+ patients who have not developed AIDS symptoms ove a period of 2 years. (26) Other studies suggest that homeopathic medicines are useful in checking the progression of HIV infection. Most studies have established that homeopathic medicines enhance the immune function and assist the infected organism to react more vigorously.

In Lyons, France, a collaboration was conducted between researchers and homeopaths. On December 12, 1991, Professor Christian Trepo, head of the Immunology and Virology Department at Hotel Dieu

Hospital in Lyons, organized a meeting of officials, researchers and 100 homeopathic physicians from the city. (27) At this meeting, Dr. Trepo stated the need to integrate non-conventional medicine to deal with the AIDS epidemic. All surveys shared at the meeting showed that a large number (35 perrcent) of HIV+ patients in French hospitals spontaneously choose alternative or unconventional medical practices, especially homeopathy, to control their conditions. At that same meeting, Professor Trepo announced that a special budget would be dedicated to integrate homeopathic physicians into his department in the hospital. Dr. Trepo became interested in homeopathic treatments for HIV/AIDS when he observed the successful results of a colleague, Dr. Jean-Bernard Carpanne, in a homeopathic clinic set up for patients with hepatitis and severe gastric disorders at Hotel Dieu Hospital.

Under a directive from the Indian Government, the Central Council for Research in Homeopathy (CCRH), has been conducting a study of 112 asymptomatic HIV+ patients since May of 1989, in Bombay. Of these patients, 12 were found to be non-reactive to ELISA on 2 or more different occasions after being treated 3-16 months. (29) The initial conclusions drawn from the study indicate that homeopathic medicines such as Syphilinum, Tuberculinum and Phosphorus may prove useful in the treatment of asymptomatic HIV+ patients.

AIDS patients are increasingly utilizing herbal medicines to alleviate certain AIDS-related symptoms and opportunistic infections. In a survey of AIDS patients conducted at a clinic of the Department of Medicine at the University of California at San Francisco, Dr. Kassler and Dr. Greenblatt discovered that 33 percent of the patients reported using one or more herbal medicines within the past three months of the time of the survey. Drs. Kassler and Greenblatt were able to identify 29 medicinal herbs that were being taken by these patients. (31) One of the concerns raised by the authors of this study is that patients often do not disclose to their primary physicians their use of alternative treatments. The lack of disclosure of the use of alternative medications, especially those enrolled in a clinical trials could distort the results of the clinical trial.

Conclusion

There continues to be very little documentation and funding of clinical studies regarding the efficacy of homeopathic medicines in the treatment of HIV/AIDS. However, Dr. Standish and other health practitioners have concluded that the compelling clinical results indicate the need for more clinical trials and research. With the establishment of the Office of Alternative Medicine at the National Institutes of Health (NIH), there is an acknowledgment by the government that a growing portion of the general population is seeking and utilizing alternative treatments. Support for research on the efficacy of homeopathic medicines in HIV/AIDS must become this office's highest priority.

Notes

1) Ullman, Dana, *Homeopathy: Medicine for the 21st Century*. Berkeley, California: North Atlantic Books, 1988, p. 22.

2) Ibid., p. 6.

3) American Institute of Homeopathy (AIH), *Standards of Homeotherapeutic Practice*, approved by AIH members, June 1985.

4) Ullman, Dana, op. cit., p. 136.

5) Ibid.

6) Ibid., p. 43.

7) Ibid.

8) Ibid., p. 40

9) Ibid., p. 41.

10) Ibid.

11) Ibid., p. 37.

12) Ibid., p. 38.

13) Ibid., p. 44

14) Ibid.

15) Ibid.

16) Ibid., p. 12

17) Ibid.

18) Ibid.

19) Kleijnen, J., et. al., "Clinical Trials of Homeopathy," *BMJ*, Vol 302, 1991, pp. 316-23.

20) Ullaman, Dana, op. cit.

21) American Institute of Homeopathy, op. cit.

22) Ullman, Dana, op. cit.

23) Ibid., p. 134.

24) Badgley, Lawrence E. "Homeopathy for Acquired Immune Deficiency Syndrome (AIDS)." The American Institute of Homeopathy, 1987.

25) Ibid.

26) Ibid.

27) Montfort, Thierry. "AIDS, Hospitals and Homeopathy," *Resonance*, 1992, pp. 5-6.

28) Ibid.

29) Rastogi, D.P., and Singh, V.P., "Human Immunodeficiency Virus (HIV) Infection, Including AIDS: Does Homeopathy Have a Role To Play in its Treatment?" *CCRH Quarterly Bulletin*, Vol. 13 (1&2), 1991.

30) Dey, S., "AIDS in India and Homeopathy," *CCRH Quarterly Bulletin*, Vol. 13 (1&2), 1991.

31) Kassler, W.J., P. Blanc, R. Greenblatt, "The Use of Medicinal Herbs by Human Immunodeficiency Virus-Infected Patients," *Archives of Internal Medicine*, Vol. 151, November 1991.

Phytotherapy: A European Approach to the Treatment of AIDS

Summary

Botanical medicine in Western Europe, particularly in France, has been influenced by the notion of "terrain," which is a generic term referring to the tissue fluids of the body, which are the cells' environment. The terrain is understood in global and qualitative terms, which implies a whole-system approach to diagnosis and treatment. Physicians in France use both Oriental and Western models as approaches to understanding the patient's clues, which point to an individualized diagnosis. Although a patient may be diagnosed as HIV positive, the actual individual condition of the patient may be far more complex. The use of essential oils plays a central role in treatment.

Principles of Aromatherapy

Aromatherapy (Phytotherapy) is the branch of botanical medicine concerned with the therapeutic use of essential oils, which are also known as "aromatics." Aromatics are administered externally through skin, orally, and even rectally, but are seldom injected, because they inherently posses great penetrating power.

Essential oils are used for their penetrating power, for their ability to treat infections, and to influence the nervous, immune and endocrine systems of the body. The disinfecting microbicidal effects of essential oils have been known to conventional science for over a century. Oil of clove, for example, has been known to have disinfecting powers 8 times stronger than phenol or carbolic acid. Oil of thyme is 13 times stronger than phenol.

Studies have been performed *in vitro* (i.e., in the Petri dish), which have shown how powerful certain oils are in killing certain bacteria and fungi. Many essential oils are much stronger than antibiotics for killing bacteria.

Beginning in the late 1960s, doctors in France began to discover some interesting phenomena. They were attempting to find out which essential oils killed which bacteria. They found many oils that had powerful effect on killing many disease-causing microbes. When a patient was suffering from a disease thought to be caused by a certain microbe, they used oils that had killed that microbe *in vitro,* or outside the body. Sometimes these oils had no effect on the patient.

In aromatherapy, the concept of the "Doctrine of the Terrain," states that the microbe is not the cause of the disease. The cause of the disease is the deteriorated internal environment, and the microbe, along with the disease symptoms, is a result of this negative environment, not the cause of it. Killing the microbe becomes incidental to the desirable therapeutic result, which actually is to restore a healthy internal milieu for the cells that live in this terrain. This terrain is not defined in terms of the microbes, which live in it, but in terms of the patient's personal characteristics. A person might have a terrain that is described as sympathicotonic-hyperthyroid, which would be an active, thin, excitable type of individual with an entire physiology, pathology and medical history typical of this nervous system profile. Doctors with Oriental training (many doctors in France are acupuncturists) might call this same person a Wood Yin individual, who has tight muscles, hyperactive nervous system, digestive sensitivity and other typical Liver symptoms. The goal of treatment, then is to correct the terrain, even in cases which require disinfection.

The observations made by doctors in France were the result of experiments that elucidated another striking phenomenon: the effective dosage of essential oils to a patient with an infection were minuscule compared to the dose required to control a microbe infection *in vitro*. To treat an internal infection, 1/100th of the dose was required of the amount necessary to kill microbes externally.

Conventional antibiotics often require large doses because they kill microbes by direct contact. Essential oils used internally do not seem to kill microbes by direct contact. They seem to alter the terrain, so that it becomes an inhospitable environment in which undesirable microbes cannot survive. Several theories were proposed to attempt to explain how this occurs. But, the theories that have not changed are those that describe the way oils are prescribed in practice, i.e., according the the patient's *typology.*

Essential Oils in Treating Infections

In terrain doctrine theory, symptoms are outward signs of disequilibrium in the internal environment. If a patient presents a case of bronchitis, the treatment strategy is not to use "bronchitis oils." Likewise, the choice of oils does not depend on whether they have properties for killing pneumococcus, streptococcus, micrococcus or staphylococcus. What might work in the isolation of a glass tray in a laboratory does not necessarily work in a complex living organism. The treatment strategy is to choose oils that match the patient's individual profile. For a patient who is "vagotonic" (tends toward excessive parasympathetic nervous system activity), oil of thyme would be an obvious choice because it is a pulmonary antiseptic and is "vagolytic," or has parasympathetic nervous system calming effects. A patient who is "hypoadrenal" (fatigued with depleted adrenal gland), might be given oil of pine, which is a pulmonary antiseptic and an adrenal cortex stimulant.

The patient could also be evaluated according to Oriental criteria. An asthma patient could be diagnosed as a "Wood Yang" with lots of "Wind-Heat," tight diaphragm, allergic symptoms but also with a Wood-Yang type of build and temperament. This patient could receive different treatment from a weak, thin, frail, exhausted Metal-Yin patient with swollen lymph nodes in the neck. herbs or oils can be classified as Wood-Yang, Metal-Yin, Water-Yin. These same herbs can be classified as sympatholytic, hypothyroid or hyperglycemiant, depending upon which diagnosis and treatment model the practitioner uses. Therefore, a single oil, such as rosemary, can be classified as Wood-Yin and Water-Yin, according to the five elements. It is also parasympathomimetic and adrenal cortex-stimulating, according to the neuro-endocrine classification model. No matter which model, the infection itself is not being treated in an of itself or to have any separate meaning or significance from the individual profile.

The Aromatogram

The aromatogram is a diagnostic test adapted from a conventional medical test called the antibiogram. A sample of the patient's sputum, urine or other discharge is cultured in the center of a Petri dish. The culture medium is surrounded by a circumference of different essential oils. Within 24 hours, it is possible to observe which oils this "terrain specimen" growing in the Petri dish likes and dislikes, by observing the direction in which it grows. if it grows in the direction away from oil of cinnamon and oil of oregano, we can safely assume that these two oils are likely to have strong therapeutic properties for that patient's terrain.

The aromatogram revealed some interesting phenomena: the same type of microbe might appear in tests from different patients but would react differently in each aromatogram. It was not the microbe that was affected by the oil, but the terrain. In other words, the sensitivity of a microbe to essential oils is not a function of the microbe itself but a function of the host organism. The most effective essential oils were also often not those that had the reputation of being strong antiseptics.

With this new tool, practitioners of phytotherapy found themselves able to effectively treat patients with persistent and intractable problems. The aromatogram is a unique diagnostic tool. It gives a qualitative rather than a quantitative evaluation of the patient's condition.

The Aromatogram and Terrain

The aromatogram provides information to assist us in understanding the complexity of the patient's condition on its own terms. The conventional notion of the AIDS patient, for example, is that the infection is caused by the HIV virus. To kill the virus is the resulting treatment strategy. The type of warfare represented by attempting to eradicate microbe populations within a living organism results in damage to the filed the battle: the patient's body. The terrain is not a metaphor for a battlefield on which invaders are destroyed. Terrain is a medium in which living creatures are nourished and cultivated. The medium will grow life according to its nature. A toxic environment grows scavengers. The cause of AIDS (the HIV virus) is an assumption that is inconsistent with the notion of biological individuality. And, the principle of biological individuality is intrinsic to the concept of the terrain.

The large, long-ignored population of HIV-positive people who are not immune deficient is an example of the concept of biological individuality and the concept of terrain. If the terrain is healthy, the patient is healthy. The presence of any type of microbe does not truly define a pathological process. The second example which comes to mind is the fact that AIDS patients don't appear to die from large reservoirs of viral overgrowth. Fungal and parasitic infections frequently play a prominent role in mortality. The whole complex of fungal and parasitic disease conditions that comprise the AIDS complex are a sizable menagerie of pathogens. The mutability of the virus, i.e., its numerous subtypes, also points to the fact that each individual grows his or her own unique ecosystem. Because of this, the aromatograms of different AIDS patients show different patterns of development and require diverse combinations of substances for treatment.

Synergistic Model of the Terrain Based on Models of Oriental Medicine and the Neuroendocrine System

A combined model of both Oriental concepts and the conventional neuroendocrine physiological model has advantages for the practitioner who takes the time to integrate these two models. Both systems contain methods of observing and accounting for a patient's individual physiological activity. The neuroendocrine model is an anatomical model, in that its components correspond to anatomically distinct structures within the body: the two branches of the autonomic nervous system and the endocrine glands. The Oriental models, on the other hand, define even anatomical structures in terms of their function. The "Heart" itself may be an actual organ, but its range of associations include memory, distinctness of speech and laughter. The Oriental model also associates a distinct topography of associated points on the arms, ears and hands.

Classifying plant substances in this way helps to describe the complexity of a plant substance. If a patient is extremely anxious, suffers insomnia, has a rapid heart rate, is flushed and chattering nervously, we would be more inclined to prescribe lavender for

Fire, rather than sweet balm (Melissa oficinalis). Sweet balm, which is Earth, would be more appropriate for the anxious patient with nausea or digestive spasms and gas. Both lavender and sweet balm are classified as sympatholytic, which means to calm excessive sympathetic nervous system activity. However, the difference in the range of associations of Fire and Earth help us to distinguish their properties. To classify and oil or herb as sympatholytic, assists in diagnosing other signs, such as the blood pressure, the type of muscle tension, the part of an organ involved in the patient's pathology or any other type of autonomic nervous system activity.

Essential Oils for AIDS Patients

Because clinical aromatherapy trials are still in early stages, there is no available data from controlled studies. This data should be available within the next year. Based on the ideas and experience of leading practitioners, there are several essences that are thought to hold great promise. These essences usually are taken orally, by inhaler, externally and rectally with a pharmaceutical quality grade of essential oil.

Oil of savory (Satureia montana) is noted as an adrenal cortex stimulant. By strengthening the adrenal cortex function, the anti-inflammatory capability of the entire system is strengthened. This is one reason that savory has long been considered a general tonic. It is particularly useful in controlling microbe populations, even protozoa. It is recognized as an antifungal, antiviral and antibacterial (including staphylococcus). There are other indications for savory's potential usefulness in AIDS. It has been used successfully for intestinal worms and to stop diarrhea. In addition to its cerebral stimulant actions, it also has been used to treat various types of skin infections.

Oil of cinnamon (Cinnamomum zeylanicum or C. cassia) and oil of clove (Eugenia caryphylata) are both used to strengthen adrenal cortex function and to stop infections. Oil of cinnamon is one of the strongest agents for treating intestinal parasites. Oil of clove is used to treat memory loss, depression and fatigue.

Oil of sage is a cerebral tonic, stimulates the secretion of pituitary hormones (gonadoptophins). It is a remarkable astringent for treating nightsweats, even in cases of pulmonary tuberculosis. It also strengthens deficient immunity and is used to treat lymph stasis, splenomegaly and chronic bronchitis.

Using Essential Oils in Combined Therapy

In early treatment and intermittently throughout, "drainage" herbs are used to clear up or prevent the buildup of a toxic burden to any of the organs, in particular the organs of elimination. Cathartics are used for the bowel, diuretics of different types are used to assist the kidneys and unburden the joints or connective tissue. Cholagogues are used to drain the bile ducts and to unburden the liver. Herbs for pancreatic drainage are used to unburden the digestive system. Herbs for lymphatic drainage are used to clear up chronic infections and to boost immunity.

Symptomatic treatment is used to relieve the energetic strain on the system, which is trying to cope with pain or with other inconvenience. Herbs used to relieve cough, pain, difficulty in sleeping, anxiety, loss of appetite, greatly assist in the healing process.

Treatment of the terrain usually involves matching the herbs to the patient's typology. It also involves chosing herbs that satisfy as many criteria as possible for drainage, symptomatic relief and to match the entire complex of the patient's symptom and sign presentation with plant substances that have harmonizing characteristics.

The symptom and sign complexes typical in AIDS are treated with herbs that simultaneously have a strengthening and gently draining effect. St. John's Wort (Hypericum perforata) among European botanicals has received much attention in the United States for its immune enhancing effects. It has been used a long time for the treatment of intestinal worms, for depression and as a general tonic. Elecampane (Inula helenium) often is used for respiratory infections but also generally stimulates pituitary function. Gentian (Gentiana lutea) dries up excessive secretions in the gastrointestinal tract and elevates white blood cell production. Fenugreek (Trigonella foenum-graecum) dries up phlegm in the respiratory and digestive tracts, strengthens adrenal cortex function, and is used to treat an underweight condition caused by malnutrition.

Herbs for treating stomatitis from candidiasis include oak bark, blue mallow and eyebright, with oils of geranium, lemon or sage. Herbs and oils, of course, are selected according to their individual properties and according to the overall picture of the terrain.

A number of herbs are used for different manifestations of herpes. However, some of the most important are herbs for drainage of the liver (such as artichoke and milk thistle) and for the skin, such as burdock and sarsaparilla. Useful essential oils include thyme, cypress, lavender, lemon, clove and geranium.

For hepatitis B, herbs for enhancing liver function are the most important: artichoke, milk thistle and oils of lemon, rosemary and geranium.

Treatment of tuberculosis has been successful with the use of many botanical substances. Among the most renowned are garlic, elecampane, fenugreek, angelica and horsetail. Among the most important essences are lemon, eucalyptus, niaouli (Melaleuca quinquenervia), clove, hyssop, lavender, pine sage and thyme.

Several botanicals have been recommended in the treatment of Kaposi's sarcoma, pneumocystis carinii pneumonia and cryptosporidiosis:

Kaposi's sarcoma: black walnut, burdock, sarsaparilla, oils of sassafras, sage, geranium and thyme.

Pneumocystis: horseradish, fenugreek, elecampane, oils of niaouli, myrtle, clove, savory, sage, lemon.

Cryptosporidiosis: black walnut, gentian, plantain, blessed thistle, oils of savory, thyme, geranium, clove, oregano, niaouli.

For anxiety and depression, angelica, milk thistle, blessed thistle, fenugreek, hypericum and bladderwrack could be used. Among the oils, essences of lavender, rosemary, savory, thyme, hyssop, basil and marjoram—all can be helpful according to each individual patient's symptoms.

Precautions

In general, the use of aromatics and plant extracts is extremely safe in comparison with most types of conventional therapy. The main precaution with the AIDS patient is to start with a small dose, so that detoxification does not occur too rapidly. Rapid detoxification can weaken patients who tend toward diarrhea or profuse sweating. Nourishing treatments such as nutritional therapy and strengthening glandular and nervous functions should always precede and accompany detoxification.

A typical daily dosage of essential oils used internally is in a range between 1 and 5 drops, one to three times a day. For an AIDS patient, 1 drop of oil of cinnamon or clove per day may be an adequate starting dose. Oil of savory or thyme could be started at a higher dose and gradually increased.

When essences are used over a long period of time or if there are certain pathological tendencies in the patient, there are several other considerations. For short-term crisis management, i.e., four to five days, there is usually no problem with any of the commonly used oils. Some of the general precautions concerning the use of essential oils include the following:

- Use lavender with caution in patients taking anticoagulants.
- If there are hard tumors, particularly of the breast, prolonged use of strongly estrogen-like oils should be avoided. Plant extracts generally have a normalizing effect on the terrain. But, long-term

use should be avoided if there is a strong endocrine effect. The most estrogenic oils include sage, cypress, angelica, fennel, anise and cumin.

- In hypothyroidism, avoid long-term use of garlic, fennel or cumin.
- In prostate cancer, avoid long-term use of wild thyme (Thymus serpyllum), cypress, angelica or hyssop.
- If there are ulcers in the digestive tract or digestive upset, restrict the use of cinnamon and clove.
- If there is high blood pressure, restrict hyssop and lemon to short-term use.
- With epilepsy, avoid sage, hyssop, fennel, parsley, nutmeg or anise.
- With urinary infections, avoid juniper and eucalyptus.
- Hot (phenolic) oils like cinnamon, clove, oregano, etc., should be used externally with caution. They can be used in small amounts with other essences in a massage oil base.
- Use only pharmaceutical grade oils for internal use. See references at the end of this article.

Of course, it is always preferable to err on the side of caution. There is very little possibility of damage or danger to the patient when essential oils are used, especially when they are used short-term for infections and anxiety attacks. The most effective use of essential oils is by understanding the terrain of the patient and matching it with the characteristics of the essences and other plant substances.

Conclusion

Botanical treatment of AIDS requires us to think qualitatively about altering the terrain to an internal environment that has greater integrity for maintaining overall vital function. It is necessary to restore endocrine function and to relieve lymph stasis gently, so that overburdened eliminative organs are not further damaged. A quantitative approach of attempting to overwhelm a population of pathogenic microbes with a "magic bullet," or any quasi-militaristic approach of attempting to destroy and invader in the form of an HIV virus or any other normal inhabitant of a pathological terrain, will be doomed to failure.

Strengthening the immune system's resources is decisive to the success of any treatment. In the case of AIDS, the use of botanicals and, in particular, aromatic essential oils, merits further investigation. This is not only because of their usefulness in controlling and neutralizing infections but also because they have such a potent effect of altering the terrain in a healthy direction rapidly and reliably.

References

Botanical Medicine: A European Perspective, Dan Kenner L.Ac., Yves Requena, M.D., Paradigm Publications.

Acupuncture et Phytothérapie, Yves Requena, M.D., Maloine S.A., Paris.

Cahiers de Phytothérapie Clinique, Duraffourd, Lapraz et d'Hervicourt, Masson, Paris.

Aromathérapie, J. Valnet, Maloine S.A., Paris.

Pour un Bon Usage des Plantes, Dr. Alain Carillon, Editions Vie & Santé, Dammarie les Lys, France.

For pharmaceutical grade essential oils, contact Ormed, Inc., PO Box 1021, Forestville, CA 95436.

The Role of Nutrition

It was assumed for many years that the role of nutrition in HIV and AIDS was at best superfluous, at worse, a waste of time and money spent on what was considered to be a terminal disease. Now, we read about how there is long-term survival in persons with HIV or AIDS due to early nutritional intervention. Many are realizing that AIDS can be (and has already become) a chronic illness, not unlike a chronic fatigue syndrome or cancer, which demand a constant attention to nutrition. Chronic illnesses are like a roller coaster ride. There are good days and bad days. To balance out those good days and bad days, it is important to adhere to daily health routines that are crucial to maintaining the regularity or homeostasis of our bodies.

We know that there are physical, emotional, psychological and biological contributors to the progressive degeneration and eventual death of cells. We also know that we can create through nutrition a fortified immune system that can ward off possible infections. At the very least, when the body does succumb to these infections, the system will have the strength and stamina through nutrient building blocks to fight infections with some greater degree of resiliency.

Our bodies are designed to be miracle machines. They undertake every conceivable function as if by magic, silently and quietly. They are a universe unto themselves. They perform millions of functions unbeknownst to us, so that we can survive in the world, seeing, hearing, thinking, moving and generally living in our surroundings as we choose. Our perception allows us to be aware of what is happening almost before it happens. Our hearing allows us to listen. our vision allows us to see. Our mouth allows us to eat and drink. Our intestines allow us to digest and utilize foods. Our colon allows us to eliminate toxins and waste by-products. Our skin allows us to prevent entry of foreign bodies.

Without thinking, we are able to function at the highest level of survival. We reflexively pull away from what is hot or jump away when we are startled. The one thing that is crucial to our survival that we must consciously do is eat. Food is the fuel that our bodies depend on to grow, to thrive, to carry on the myriad of functions that are required to keep our bodies active and alert.

We know that food is important because of what we nutritionally derive from it. Protein, carbohydrates and fats are made in the body. But, these nutrients are made mostly by synthesizing building blocks of these materials from what we eat. Vitamins and minerals are crucial because our bodies do not synthesize them. However, they are essential to the system. They serve at different levels of biochemical reactions, mostly as co-enzymes in metabolic functions. They turn on and speed along chemical reactions at every level. Vitamins and minerals are present in any biological reaction in the body, from the uptake and utilization of glucose to the production of ATP for energy.

From the early studies of vitamin C, when it was discovered that a deficiency of it caused scurvy, we have been fascinated with the role of nutrients in food. People who ate limes didn't develop scurvy and those who did not eat limes developed scurvy.

Although this relationship seemed simple, it was limited to a traditional point of view that "health is the absence of disease." This traditional point of view asked, "what is the least amount of nutrient required to prevent disease?"However, if we move beyond the limited traditional viewpoint to ask, "what is the amount of nutrient to ensure optimal health and function?" we reach a completely different answer.

In a condition such as AIDS, when the body is in a distress situation and responding to an emergency alert state, there is an increase in the metabolic rate. The body is trying to return to a state of homeostasis. This can be seen during infections, fevers and even stress syndromes, when the body literally is working overtime to promote cell production during rapid cell turnover and cell death. The body requires an increase in the nutrient building blocks (amino acids, polysaccharides, fatty acids, etc.) in order to continue providing higher energy requirements.

From international studies done over the past 10-20 years, we have learned much about nutrition and malnutrition. Much of what we see with classic malnutrition is similar to findings at various stages of AIDS, such as weight loss, diarrhea, gastro-intestinal dysbiosis and loss of appetite. Although it is important to identify the cause of the problem, nutritionally speaking, it is more important to arrest the symptoms. One study compared the outcome of the most expensive diagnostic testing with no testing at all. The subjects were ultimately treated identically, with psyllium fiber to bulk up the stool and delay the transit time. What they discovered was that at the treatment itself was crucial. With diarrhea, the very danger lies in losing important nutrients, especially minerals, which contribute to electrolyte loss and possible death.

The main emphasis in AIDS research has been to find the magic bullet cure: the one drug or vaccine that will eradicate the HIV virus, which is believed to be the sole cause of AIDS. As research and rethinking of AIDS has continued, what we are seeing is more evidence that other factors are involved. It is becoming more apparent that the breakdown of the immune system is from more than one virus, bacteria or parasite. It appears that there can be a number of co-factors that can substantially contribute to the weakening of the immune system. If we shift our focus and emphasize the "whole" system and relinquish the war on one solitary virus, we can then work on ensuring that the body remains in a homeostatic state through optimal nutrition.

We know that through proper nutrient intake, we can reverse malnutrition. Malnutrition leads to many immune compromising failures in the body. Besides weight loss, diarrhea, gastro-intestinal disorders and loss of lean muscle mass, there are decreased white blood cell production, anemia, fatigue, exhaustion and lowered resistance to fight off infections. Instead of waiting for degeneration through malnutrition to occur in AIDS, a preventative approach of aggressive treatment through early nutritional intervention is necessary. If the system has the available stamina, energy and nutrient building blocks when it requires them, it at least will be fortified to ward off and prevent infections and other disease processes.

Studies indicate that long term survivors of AIDS generally take better care of their bodies, their minds and their spirits. Although we all would like to be able to provide these nutrients through food alone, the reality is that most foods lack true nutritive value to sustain even healthy individuals. Environmental toxins, tainted water supplies, pesticides, xenobiotics, mineral depleted soils, prolonged shipping time, processing, refinement, and cooking of foods. All of these factors contribute to vitamin and mineral loss. Individuals who are immune compromised are even less able to overcome these environmental vitamin and mineral losses than healthy individuals.

In any condition of health, it essential to strengthen the immune system functioning through choosing high quality foods that provide protein, carbohydrates, fat and high calories. High calories alone without these other essential nutrients will not be sufficient. Some foods can provide immediate enhancement of immune function. Other foods demand more energy from the body to break them down than they actually provide to the system. Some foods can generate high energy as measured by calories, but they cannot provide high quality nutrients.

Following are lists of foods to avoid and foods to eat for individuals with HIV infection and AIDS.

Foods To Avoid

Refined White Flour and Sugars

These over-processed foods provide no nutritive value and clog the system. They break down too rapidly into glucose, which overtaxes the pancreas, adrenals and liver. They also lack vitamins, minerals and fiber.

Coffee and Caffeine-Containing Substances

Although many of these are natural stimulants, they overstress the adrenal glands and hinder the breakdown of glucagon, a stored form of glucose. They also rob the body of water soluble vitamins by increasing the body's metabolism.

Excessive Meats (Especially Red)

The body can experience difficulty in digesting heavy fats and animal proteins. Animal fats provide higher levels of inflammatory prostaglandins (PGE1). Contamination from bacteria, worms and parasites can occur when meat is undercooked. Ingesting meat from animals that are fed antibiotics and hormones and exposed to pesticides can further damage immune function.

Shellfish (Especially Raw)

Contamination from bacterial sewage, parasites and viruses can infect the body and place more stress on its immune functions.

Dairy Products

Some people cannot tolerate lactose sugar. This lactose intolerance can cause gastrointestinal upset, cramping and diarrhea. High fat dairy products can cause difficulty in digestion and increased mucous. Milk is laden with antibiotics, pesticides and hormones. Highly cultured yogurt with natural bacteria is preferable in small amounts.

Hydrogenated or Partially Hydrogenated Oils

These oils have been chemically altered (usually with heat) from liquids to create creams or hard solids (e.g., margarine, greasy fried foods, potato chips). These hydrogenated or partially hydrogenated oils are known to act as carcinogenic agents in the body.

What To Eat

The dietary emphasis for persons with HIV and AIDS is low total fat, high quality protein and high fiber. The guidelines are similar to diets, which help prevent and reverse heart disease and cancer. So, if we are placing less emphasis on meats and dairy (common to a Western diet), then what are the alternatives?

Whole Grains and Dried Beans

Whole grains provide complex carbohydrates for long-term fuel, fiber and a good source of B vitamins. Beans are a high quality protein. With whole grains, beans provide a complete protein with all of the essential amino acids, good sources of fat and fiber for long-term energy.

Nuts and Seeds

Nuts and seeds are an excellent, rich source of fiber, minerals, vitamins, protein, carbohydrate and fat.

Fresh Fruits, Vegetables and Sea Vegetables

These foods are rich in vitamins A and C, beta-carotene, calcium and many other minerals. They should be eaten in season, raw, steamed, juiced, stewed or lightly sautéed. Dried fruits should be avoided, because they are too concentrated in natural sugars and can provide a ripe environment for yeast overgrowth.

Water

Drinking at least 8 glasses of water daily assists in flushing out impurities and waste matter.

Fresh Vegetable and Fruit Juices

These fresh juices are a great source of alkaline cleansing. Most toxins in the system (i.e., drugs, alcohol, caffeine, etc.) tend to be more acidic in nature. Rebalancing with alkaline juices allows the body to flush out impurities, clear excessive mucous production and empty out fecal impaction. Diluting these juices with water decreases their high sugar concentration. Some examples of combined juices include: carrot-beet-celery, papaya-pineapple-mango, avocado-papaya, kale-parsley-carrot, watermelon-apple-grape. Garlic and ginger also are good additions.

Soybean and Brown Rice Products

These foods are excellent replacements for dairy and are a good source of protein, calcium and fiber. Their nutrients can be obtained in various forms: tofu cakes, yogurt, milk, ice cream and creamy dressings.

Fresh Fish

Fresh fish is a great source of omega-2 essential fatty acids, which are necessary for prostaglandin production. PGE2 is a very important prostaglandin, because it acts as an anti-inflammatory agent. Fish also is a good source of protein, vitamins A and D, and minerals.

Free-Range Chicken

Free-range chicken is hormone and antibiotic free. It is a good source of protein and some B vitamins. It is lower in animal fat and, if limited to 4-ounce servings, it is easier to digest than factory-produced chicken.

Fats and Oils

Flaxseed oil is the best vegetarian combination source of the omega-3 (linoleic acid), the omega-6 (linolenic acid) and the omega-9 (oleic acid) essential fatty acids. They are essential because the body does not produce them. They are necessary for many crucial functions, such as prostaglandin production, insuring smooth muscle arterial blood flow, nerve transmission, etc. The most active form of omega-3 is derived from fish liver oils. Omega-6 is abundant in borage oil, black currant seed oil and, to a lesser extent, evening primrose oil. Fatty acids are important to transport fat soluble vitamins, store energy, produce energy, make hormones, cushion and protect organs. Some polyunsaturated oils are: safflower, sunflower, soybean and corn. Some monosaturated oils (for the production of HDL cholesterol) are olive and canola.

Size and Frequency of Meals

Eating smaller, more frequent meals makes it easier to digest the food properly. It also allows a moderate breakdown and uptake of glucose during digestion. This moderate breakdown and absorption of glucose creates a continuous source of energy over longer periods of time.

Macrobiotic Diets

In theory, macrobiotics is the harmonizing of certain foods eaten in the region and the season in which they were grown. It is a balancing of the Yin and Yang energy. This balancing is symbolized by a coin. Yin and Yang are the sides of the same coin. In Chinese and Japanese systems, this is called "what is within is without." Qi is the internal energy that we harness from outside us to inside us. Yin and Yang foods are taken in balance to promote Qi. Yin foods tend to be more alkaline in nature. They generally are the fruits and vegetables. Yin represents the "softer, more feminine" side, associated with fall and winter. Yang foods tend to be more acidic in nature. They are the grains and protein foods. Yang represents the "harder, more masculine" side of the coin. It is associated with more expansive seasons of spring and summer.

For example, in a Yin season (winter), Yang (grains and protein are usually taken to expand (heat) from the contraction (cold.) Conversely, in a Yang (summer) season, more fruits and vegetables are eaten to contract (cold) from the expansion (heat).

In theory, the balancing of foods in this manner is ideal. In practice, however, people tend to become too severe in their choice of foods. Some choose only brown rice and some vegetables, which can do more harm than good. Many problems can arise when there is improper balancing of nutrients. There may be insufficient protein intake or insufficient caloric intake to meet an individuals higher metabolic needs. A particular problem is presented when there is no intake of animal products at all, especially dairy, which can contribute to a vitamin B 12 deficiency.

A macrobiotic diet can be ideal when used as a cleansing diet and when followed as a general guideline to eating. Some people do not do well physically as strict vegetarians and would be better off adding small amounts of animal products. Others have found that a rice based protein can be a good substitute. The crucial determining point must be the maintenance of lean muscle mass and body weight. It must be emphasized that the immune compromised patient is at risk of protein malnourishment. This inadequate protein intake can leas to wasting syndrome, diarrhea and weight loss.

If an individual's weight is stable and can do well on a strict vegetarian diet, then this diet should be continued. However, it is advisable to supplement this diet with high calorie protein shakes, which can further augment both protein and calorie intake.

Nutrients and Supplements for the Treatment of HIV/AIDS

The other important recommendation would be to vary foods and to utilize supplement nutrients in the treatment of HIV/AIDS.

Some of these supplements would include: anti-oxidants, botanical and anti-viral therapy, minerals, vitamins, herbs, glandulars and homeopathic remedies.

Nutrient Therapy: The DAAIR Protocol

DAAIR

Direct AIDS Alternative Information Resources (DAAIR) is a non-profit organization formed to promote self-empowered healing from HIV disease through the use of natural therapies (particularly nutrients) and minimally toxic drugs. Central to this approach is a perspective which allows for strategic immune supports and a strengthening of the body's own abilities (host defense) to fight chronic, ongoing infection.

People with HIV (PWHIVs), who have organized DAAIR, have intensively researched the scientific literature, consulted physicians and other PWHIVs, and experimented on themselves to develop state-of-the-art recommended protocols of treatments, which are updated periodically. The centerpiece of this approach is a mulitfactorial model and a group of substances known generally as antioxidant nutrients to combat the oxidative stress (caused by excess of damaging "free-radical" molecules), which creates and environment for HIV disease to progress. DAAIR not only supplies information on these therapies but also runs a Buyers Club, which uses bulk purchasing and moral persuasion to make these therapies affordable to members.

The DAAIR Buyers Club offers lower prices on its products and provides an information source for PWHIVs. The membership fee to join the club is $5 and includes an introductory 150+-page packet, which explains, in lay language, the logic and science supporting the various parts of its recommended nutrient therapy protocols. DAAIR also holds other public information meetings.

DAAIR neither endorses nor prescribes any particular treatment. All members are strongly encouraged to regularly discuss their treatment program with a knowledgeable health professional. DAAIR does not assume any responsibility or liability for any adverse effects or consequences resulting from the sale or use of any product provided by DAAIR or described in any of DAAIR's informational materials.

Nutrient Therapy

Nutrients are simply the chemical components in food that nourish or build up the body. Studies have shown that the from the onset of HIV infection, all people have multiple deficiencies of critical nutrients. Supplementing these nutrients, the building blocks of life, if done in sufficient dosages, can exert profoundly beneficial and healing effects on the body.

Nutrients that are used in the DAAIR protocols include: amino acids antioxidants, minerals, fatty acids, helpful bacteria, glandular products, herbal extracts and prescriptive medicines—all of which have been shown in research to strengthen the immune system, slow viral growth and aid in the defense against chronic illness. This parallels an increasing trend in many countries towards acceptance of alternative healing practices. One recognition of this development is the recent establishment of a small Office of Alternative Medicine at the National Institutes of Health to begin to evaluate scientific studies of these complementary approaches to health.

Therapeutic Goals for Persons with HIV

1) To slow increasing production of oxidants and to restore the body's natural balance of antioxidants. Oxidants are unstable pieces of molecules, called "free radical, "which easily react with and harm intact cells in the body. Antioxidants are compounds which easily give up parts of themselves to protect against damage to the body. By reestablishing this oxidative imbalance, the immune system is made stronger, while viruses inside cells become less active. This slows disease progression as well as the autoimmune component (the body's mistaken attack on its own cells), which clearly develops as HIV progresses.

2) To restore critical sulfur amino acids (cysteine, glutathione, methionine), which prevents early apoptosis (the self-destruction of immune cells that have lost their glutathione). Glutathione itself is the critical amino acid that regulates the cell cycle, the birth and death and viral production of infected cells. Restoration of sulfur amino acids (the building blocks of protein) also slows syncitcia (the clumping together and destruction of immune cells), stops excessive releases of other inflammatory products ("free radicals") and other product naturally produced in the immune

response to kill foreign invaders. It is well documented that HIV virus pieces, which increase in the body as the virus grows, are themselves severe oxidants.

3) To reverse critical nutrient deficiencies, which are common, even in early HIV infection, and which quicken disease progression. A constant, ongoing and deteriorating HIV infection, along with a chronic immune response, places specific, well-documented, early nutrient drains on the body (A, B-2, B-6, B-12, C, E, zinc, selenium and copper) In full-blown AIDS, nearly every nutrient is deficient.

4) To improve intestinal health. It is well-documented that even in early HIV infection, the gut immune cells are not working properly and allow for easy infection and malabsorption (the poor uptake of nutrients). This HIV-induced malnutrition can only speed disease progression.

5) To provide direct antivirals with little cumulative toxicity (the increasing toxic build-up in the body by pharmaceuticals). There are many natural compounds, particularly plant products (licorice, garlic, bitter melon), which can directly and naturally interfere with HIV's ability to replicate and to enter into cells without developing resistance (the virus' ability to change to avoid a particular drug). These varied substances also slow the infection of other lipid (fat) coated organisms, which act as co-factors (infection which join together with HIV to speed immune cell loss).

6) To provide generally immune-supportive and normalizing substances that help the body fight chronic infections without adding to the autoimmune components, or increasing

inflammation or immune dysregulation (the abnormal production and processing of immune cell information), which creates further disease progression.

7) To strengthen the entire physical and mental body, the host defense, which lives as an interrelated and complete system of balanced and connected parts. This strengthening can be achieved through the use of therapeutic substances with low toxicities, including nutrients and herbs. These substances traditionally have been know and used to support overall body functions and increase its ability to fight disease in a biologically sustainable and naturally supportive manner.

Vitamins and Minerals

Comprehensive Vitamin/Mineral Supplement

Research has shown that PWHIVs use 22 percent more nutrients and energy in fighting chronic viral infection than HIV negative persons. There also are well documented and specific nutrient depletions early in HIV infection. In more advanced stages of HIV, several groups of researchers report that nearly every major nutrient is deficient. Some of these nutrients, like the carotenoids and sulfur amino acids, are extremely low. Therefore, there is no question that supplementing to alleviate these deficiencies can slow disease progression and lessen some symptoms.

Researchers from the University of Miami Medical School report that nutrient deficiencies begin early in asymptomatic stages of HIV infection. These deficiencies can directly influence both the functioning of the immune system and the rate of disease progression. Other researchers both here (notably at

Yale University) and abroad have documented that correcting such deficiencies as beta-carotene, zinc, selenium, B-6 and B-12 actually resulted in T-cell increases and/or stabilization of immune functioning.

A number of studies have been concluded recently that point quite clearly to a benefit from early and sustained use of dietary supplements. In a UCLA study, B. Abrams, et. al., noted the "almost one-third of the 296 HIV-positive participants maintaining strict diet and vitamin treatments were protected from the onset of AIDS over the course of six years." With certain statistical adjustments, those who took daily multivitamin supplements were only 70 percent as likely to progress to AIDS as those who did not.

In a Johns Hopkins Medical Institutions study of 281 HIV positive men for up to 6.8 years found a 40 to 48 percent drop in progression to AIDS among the study sample. The "data suggest that micronutrient intake needs to be sustained for at least two years and started early in the infection to be most effective," concludes Neil Grahm, senior author of the paper. Research also has detailed early and increasing immune dysfunction found along the digestive tract (known to be a primary site of HIV infection in many PWHIVs), allowing for bacterial, fungal and other microbial infections which, along with other co-factors, worsen nutrient absorption.

To compensate for this malabsorption, a good multivitamin with minerals should be the cornerstone of any type of HIV protocol.

Along with microorganism-related malabsorption problems, PWHIVs also have high inflammatory (free radical-generating) immune messenger levels (cytokines) in their blood, which generate large amounts of free radicals. These free radicals are known to severely disrupt fat metabolism and create fat-soluble malabsorption. These inflammatory immune messengers are known as Tumor Necrosis Factor. Interferon-alpha, interferon-gamma and interlukin-1, among others, are found along the intestinal tract in increased amounts, even early in HIV disease. This may account for the early fat-soluble malabsorption seen in PWHIVs.

This condition is worsened by the severe body-wide deficiencies in sulfur amino acids, particularly in the cells along the intestinal tract. Sulfur amino acids in these cells would normally act as co-enzymes, facilitating absorption of many nutrients.

Comprehensive Antioxidant Supplement

Next to a multivitamin, additional levels of various antioxidants are the most critical components of any HIV treatment plan. Antioxidants are protective compounds that work in unison and synergistically (together their combined use increases each one's individual effectiveness).

Research at Dr. Luc Montaigner's Pasteur Institute as well as at a National Institutes of Health (NIH) conference has clearly shown that there is severe oxidative imbalance (an excess of free radicals and depletion of protective antioxidants) in HIV infection. This imbalance worsens as the disease progresses. Antioxidants are depleted in fighting free radicals. Free radicals are excessively generated by four types of destructive compounds and processes: HIV proteins, excess immune signaling messengers (cytokines), immune system overactivation (inflammation), and increased cellular energy production.

Free radicals are molecules with unpaired electrons (parts of the cell normally balanced in twos), which because of their instability steal electrons from other molecules, thereby damaging cells. Free radicals have been implicated in aging and in several degenerative diseases, including cancers and immune system disorders. Antioxidants also are known as free-radical scavengers because they neutralize free radicals by donating electrons.

Free radicals can have external environmental sources, such as drugs, pesticides, sunlight, x-rays, cleaning fluids, air pollution (including cigarette smoke) and certain foods (mainly fried, barbecued, additive-laden and synthetic). Free radicals can be produced internally by immune cells themselves, which either use free radicals to dissolve foreign invaders or actually shoot "bullets" of free radicals at foreign invaders or malfunctioning cells in order to destroy them. This immune process is inflammation, which can be seen as the redness, swelling and heat around an open cut, but which also spreads internally. A clear mark of HIV infection is that inflammation becomes exaggerated, generalized and dysfunctional. Parts of the immune system become locked in overdrive while other parts diminish. This process can become even more exaggerated by co-factor infections, which created further immune activation, increasing the inflammatory aspects of the immune systems as immune cells generate more free radicals in order to help fend off the foreign invader (infection). Thus, there is a generalized build-up of abnormally high levels of free-radical-generating cytokines or inflammatory immune messengers. These messengers (interferons alpha and gamma, tumor necrosis factors [TNFs] and others the immune system uses to signal its interrelated parts) and their by-products (cortisol, prostaglandins, histamines, etc.) constantly generate free radicals. Some immune cells also become directly infected with HIV, which tells the cell to produce even more of these free radical (inflammatory) immune messengers. This process of inflammatory immune dysregulation favors the increasing growth of HIV within cells because free radicals help to "turn on" and increase the growth of HIV.

Another natural source of increased free radicals is from the body's production of energy. Inside every cell is an energy producing factory. Of the energy that the individual cell produces, between 6-8 percent of that energy releases free radicals. Since PWHIVs use 22 percent more energy and nutrients fighting chronic infection, there are possibly 22 percent more free radicals created as well.

HIV proteins are themselves severely inflammatory and destructive to cells. One viral protein, called gp120 has been added to laboratory dishes with human cells and dramatically increased (up to 40 fold) the release of inflammatory by-products and free radicals. Another part of the HIV virus, called Tat, has been found to severely disrupts and deplete a critical enzyme system inside human cells called manganese SOD. This enzyme is responsible for protecting the cell against free radical accumulation by increasing the major protector against free radical accumulation, a sulfur amino acid, glutathione. In monkey models of HIV infection, glutathione dropped by over 60 percent after the first two weeks of infection with HIV and never returned to normal. This mechanism, which is used by HIV to deplete cells of free-radical-protecting compounds, makes the host cell more likely to grow HIV at a high rate.

Glutathione deficiency has been documented in humans as well as other critical sulfur amino acids (methionine and cysteine. HIV infected monkey models, which do not lose their immune system or sicken and die when infected with HIV, also never lose any of their sulfur amino acids. No one yet knows why free radical protecting sulfur amino acids drop so quickly and dramatically at the very onset of HIV infection. But, some researchers believe that it is because these very inflammatory HIV proteins initially flood the body before any antibody immune response has a chance to regain control and suppress their production.

Early HIV infection is controlled through the loss of critical sulfur amino acids. Later, the inflammatory immune dysregulation and free radicals build up and disrupt fat metabolism (the body's ability to process and manufacture certain fat-based nutrients and other products). In the early stages of HIV infection, the inflammatory immune messengers (cytokines) increase along the digestive tract. Several researchers feel that the increased cytokines at this site of nutrient absorption compromise the body's ability to utilize critical fat-soluble nutrients (vitamin A, E, beta-carotene and other carotenes, co-enzyme Q-10 and fatty acids).

As HIV infection proceeds, the oxidative imbalance (the presence of too many free radicals and too few protective antioxidants) is increased. This imbalance assures viral activation. Viruses that have already been integrated inside cells can be asleep (latent) or can replicate at a very low level until they are stimulated by free radicals. Unless this process is successfully reversed or slowed down with antioxidant supplementation, further immune dysregulations and disease progression occur.

Because of their critical role in immune regulation, many antioxidants can be considered antiviral treatments because they lessen activation of HIV and other viruses in the laboratory by inhibiting the free-radical-driven switches of the the HIV Long Terminal Repeat (LTR). LTR turns on some of the viral activation pathways. The major pathway is known as Nuclear Factor kappa B or NFkB.

Again, antioxidants work in unison and synergistically. Their combined use increases each individual effectiveness. This is why a comprehensive antioxidant supplement is recommended.

Beta-Carotene

There is a documented severe deficiency of the carotenoids in PWHIVs. Carotenoids are pre-vitamin A family of nutrients. One of the carotenoids is beta-carotene. Some physicians have begun aggressively supplement HIV treatment with high doses of this critical free radical scavenger, which also protects the outer layer of cells and thymus production.

This nutrient, along with Vitamin E and others, is a fat-soluble, which is poorly absorbed in PWHIVs. Multiple studies (including at Yale University) have shown that doses in excess of 100,000-198,000 IU in advanced HIV infection can increase CD-4 cells substantially.

In one study, presented at the Berlin AIDS Conference in 1993, 64 asymptomatic PWHIVs were given 100,000 IUs per day for 20 out of 30 days. Their T-cells increased on average by roughly 15 percent or 68 T-4 cells over a period of 21 months.

In New York City, several physicians have been administering 500,000 IU per day, taken along with soy oil to increase absorption, with little toxicity and modest immune improvements and/or stabilization over a six-month period.

Vitamin A in excess of 25,000-100,000 IU per day may be toxic to the body. Beta-carotene is preferable, since it is safely converted by the body to vitamin A as needed. There is a very low toxicity profile for larger doses of beta-carotene, except for diabetics and those with advanced liver impairments. Dosage should be reduced if an orange color develops in the palms of the hands.

Vitamin B Complex

Along with a multivitamin and antioxidant complex, a good B-complex is another essential core nutrient for PWHIVs. It has been established that several B vitamins are required in greater quantities than the Recommended Daily Dose (RDA) for PWHIVs. The B vitamins, along with vitamin C, are water soluble and easily excreted by the body in a short period of time. Therefore, they should be replenished continuously.

There are critical functions for several B vitamins in HIV infection, which can result in their depletion in the body. B-2 is used up by the increased production of several key antioxidant enzyme systems inside the cells, which utilize scarce sulfur amino acids to protect against the abnormally high levels of oxidative stress. B-2 also acts as a co-enzyme for the recycling of many other antioxidants. B-6 is responsible for the conversion of amino acids into various protein complexes. It is depleted by the overproduction of antibodies (proteins), which is common in HIV infection. B-12 possibly needs glutathione (GSH) or other sulfur based amino acids to be synthesized along the intestinal tract. All three of these B vitamins are critical to immune function in many other ways, acting as co-enzymes in a variety of other processes.

Vitamin B-6

Research has shown that replenishing the level of vitamin B-6, which is frequently substantially deficient in HIV infection, can increase T-cell levels as well as alleviate anxiety, depression and other neurological problems.

This critical B vitamin is absolutely necessary for those on TB drugs or AZT. Both of these drugs deplete vitamin B-6.

Vitamin B-12 and Folic Acid

Vitamin B-12 is a commonly deficient nutrient with multiple quality-of-life effects. Fatigue and neurological complications such as memory loss, confusion, depression, slowed mental reactions, peripheral neuropathy (numbness, pins and needles, particularly in extremities or muscle weakness) are common problems with HIV infection. Because B-12 deficiency can be a major causative factor in all of these symptoms, it is important to supplement with high doses along with a moderate amount of additional folic acid.

Unfortunately, the standard blood tests for B-12 deficiency are often inaccurate, and depletions in the tissues can occur over a year before blood levels show a significant decline. It may take over 8 weeks to replenish depleted B-12 levels. Symptoms may take time to show improvement. Serious deficiencies may be treated through a health care provider in weekly or twice-weekly shots of B-12, between 1,000-2,000 mcg. for up to 10 weeks to restore normal levels.

Some PWHIVs have reported that taking glutathione with B-12 seems to increase its absorption. There is a definite connection between the sulfur amino acids and some of the B vitamins. Particularly for those taking AZT, B-12 may very well help prevent or alleviate the occurrence of anemia and bone marrow toxicity.

Vitamin C

In any HIV protocol, vitamin C is another critical nutrient. Vitamin C is an antioxidant and highly efficient free radical scavenger, antiviral, antibacterial and antifungal. Vitamin C is responsible for the reactivation (reduction or redox) of key antioxidants, particularly vitamin E, beta-carotene and GSH, after they have been oxidized by donating electrons to neutralize a free radical. Vitamin C and certain sulfur amino acids are the only water-soluble nutrients that can be taken in sufficiently large, yet safe, quantities to effectively conduct this redox process.

Vitamin C is available in quick- and slow-release tablets, powders, as well as esterified (vitamin C chemically bonded with one or more minerals) and effervescent forms. It may be found as ascorbic acid or complexed to various minerals as ascorbates. The mineral and esterified forms of ascorbate are advantageous because they are absorbed by the body more quickly. They are also buffered, so that they are less acidic and more easily tolerated by the stomach than ascorbic acid. Laboratory studies by Jonathan Wright, M.D., found that esterified vitamin C was absorbed into white blood cells at double the level of ascorbate C (granular vitamin C with minerals) and quadruple the level of ascorbic acid (pure vitamin C).

Bioflavanoids such as Rutin and Quericitin, which coexist with ascorbic acid in nature, enhance vitamin C activity. Pycnogenol (proanthocyanidins) is a potent antioxidant bioflavanoid extracted from grape seeds.

Like the sulfur amino acids, vitamin C should be taken in a mix of different forms if economically feasible. Usual dose is between 9-20 grams per day. A good minimum combination vitamin C protocol would include 3-4 esterol per day along with 4-6 grams of ascorbic acid in either powder or pill form. Some might want to use both ascorbic and ascorbate forms together or separately. Higher doses above 20 grams per day should be tested for bowel tolerance levels. These are the levels of vitamin C intake just below the doses which cause a harmless diarrhea reaction. At this point, the optimal antiviral antioxidant levels are reached. Vitamin C above 8 grams per day never should be stopped suddenly. These doses should be reduced gradually over an extended period.

An Overview of Viral Growth and Development

The HIV virus must insert its genetic machinery into the genetic machinery of the human cell in order to grow and replicate. HIV is a retrovirus that converts RNA pieces into human DNA in order to grow. HIV uses an enzyme to do this. Enzymes are like the conveyor belts in a factory, which move and transform things. HIV uses these enzymes, called reverse transcriptase (RT) to insert its viral RNA into the human cells' DNA. RT is a very error-prone enzyme, which is 1,000 times more likely to make mistakes translating RNA to DNA than human enzymes, which normally are used by the human body to build cells from human DNA.

AZT, DDI, DDC, D4T, 3TC and the non-nucleoside reverse transcriptase inhibitors are designed to inhibit RT and partially stop the virus from integrating itself into human cells. These drugs cannot control HIV infection once the virus has used RT and translated itself into the human molecular machinery. This group of infected cells represents a substantial, even major percentage of viral activity, which already is inside the machinery of the human cell.

The Long Terminal Repeat (LTR) is the site of the virus which controls the rate and degree of viral production once HIV has incorporated itself into the cell and becomes chronically active. There are several drugs that are being developed that do not affect RT and other viral products have been translated using the highly error-prone RT enzyme. One of these drugs is the new protease inhibitor. Unfortunately, because of the 1,000 fold increase in errors creating these viral products, mutations occur in the translation of viral RNA into DNA. As these mistakes (mutations) occur and increase in number, the actual structure of the viral products changes and the drugs designed to bind to the viral surfaces no longer fit properly and become ineffective. Scientists call this "viral resistance" to the particular drug.

HIV makes 15 proteins. This is a very small amount. So, in order to grow, HIV must also use parts of the human cell (referred to as "cellular" as opposed to viral parts) in order to replicate. The good thing about these cellular components of viral growth is that they use human enzymes to be created and not RT. Therefore, they are much less likely to mutate.

Several of the cellular parts of viral activation are to be found in the LTR section of the virus, its "on/off switch." Two of these areas of the LTR, called binding sites, are for a human cell product called Nuclear Factor kappa B (NFkB). NFkB is activated by free radicals and is used in many different human cells, particularly immune cells, to activate them. NFkB is not exclusively used for the virus to activate but by different human immune cells to produce critical immune messengers (called cytokines), which the body uses as a signaling system between immune cells. Many of these immune messengers have been found to be excessively produced during HIV infection. Several of them, including Tumor Necrosis Factor (TNF), actually direct the body to produce more free radicals and are therefore called inflammatory cytokines.

When HIV creates an internal state of oxidative imbalance, this favors the overexpression of free radical activated NFkB, which forces immune cells to produce the very inflammatory products which increase viral growth. Free radicals activate NFkB, which in turn, activates not only HIV through the NFkB binding sites along the LTRR but also increases the production of free-radical-generating immune messengers (inflammatory cytokines). A viscious, self-sustaining cycle is created, called oxidative imbalance, in which the body has few antioxidant stores and many free radicals.

In a number of laboratory studies, antioxidants, which diminish free radicals, have have been shown to inhibit HIV viral growth by inhibiting NFkB along the LTR. Laboratory studies of viral inhibition have been completed for thioctic acid, vitamin E derivatives, vitamin C, glutathione (which also slows viral incorporation into acutely infected cells), NAC, pentoxyfylline (Trental), as well as the bioflavanoid quercetin. Because NFkB is a cellular product using a relatively error free enzyme, it is doubtful that viral resistance to these NFkB inhibitory compounds will develop. By slowing or stopping viral growth in chronic cells that are already infected, viral mutations to RT viral products also will be greatly slowed down.

Because these compounds either stop or slow down viral activation in chronically infected cells in which RT inhibitors are ineffective, they are, at the very least, another mechanism for slowing disease progression. Like other diseases, HIV infection probably will only be controlled with a combination of different drugs working against different areas of the virus in different virus/cell populations. We need further research on drugs that will inhibit the cellular sites (where drug resistance is unlikely to develop) of the LTR combined with protease and RT inhibitors, as well as others. So, antioxidant use represents only one part of a multifactorial combination strategy to either halt or slow down disease progression.

Vitamin E

Vitamin E belongs to a class of antivirals which, in the laboratory, inhibit a section of the virus called the Long Terminal Repeat (LTR). LTR basically is the viral on/off switch.

Next to beta-carotene, vitamin E, which is a fat-soluble antioxidant, can be difficult to absorb and is critically depleted in HIV infection. This is because of the generalized inflammatory conditions that occur with HIV infection.

Vitamin E, like other antioxidants, may be considered directly antiviral against a viral that already has been fully integrated into cells but may be asleep or replicating at a low level. Vitamin E acts to inhibit the NFkB, a cellular product that is a relatively error-free enzyme. By inhibiting NFkB in laboratory conditions, vitamin E (along with glutathione, vitamin C, NAC, quercetin and thioctic acid) are able to stop the activation of latent virus already incorporated into the cell, which the nucleosides AZT, DDI, DDC, etc., are ineffective in controlling. Once HIV has been integrated into the molecular machinery of the cell, nucleoside analogues lose their usefulness.

Research has also shown that chronically active cells which have HIV actively replicating in them can either be returned to a latent state or the level of replication can be reduced, by reducing free radicals generated inside the cells.

Like other antioxidants, vitamin E is synergistic (works together in a more powerful manner) with other antioxidants. In particular, it is recycled (returned to a state of being able to control free radicals) inside the cell by glutathione. Glutathione, in turn, is reactivated by vitamin C. This is why it is important to take a balanced combination of antioxidant substances for the greatest effect.

Important research at Tulane University revealed that vitamin E may potentiate the effectiveness of AZT and reduce bone marrow toxicity This only makes sense if vitamin E and AZT are working on different pools of virus within the body.

Minerals

Calcium phosphorus, magnesium, potassium and molybdenum are important for cell membrane integrity, cell absorption, to alleviate fatigue, muscle cramps, loss of smell and taste and many other bodily functions.

Mineral depletion in HIV infected individuals is more pronounced when taking pharmaceutical drugs used to treat HIV infection.

Selenium

This important antioxidant trace mineral (a metal found in the body in very small amounts) helps prevent free radical damage while boosting the power of vitamin E. Dosage should not exceed 800 mcg. per day.

Sulphur

Methysulfonylmethane (MSM) is a rich source of bioavailable sulfur, and indispensable element in human nutrition. Sulfur binds with a variety of toxicants through sulfur conjugation, a major detoxification pathway in the body. This process lessens a variety of allergic reactions.

MSM also has a history of use in greatly reducing chronic inflammatory pain and generalized muscle soreness, including leg and back cramps. Sulfur labeled MSM has also been found to be incorporated into protein cysteine residues throughout the body, thereby serving as a valuable secondary source for already severely depleted sulfur amino acids in HIV infection.

When it is used in food and drug allergies, it is administered in 100-1,000 mg. concurrently with the allergen or irritant. It has proven ability to reduce or eliminate such reactions. Under certain conditions, a loading dose of 2-5 grams for a period of five days may be necessary before challenge with the allergen. Please consult with a health care professional for appropriate instructions.

Zinc and Copper

Zinc has been found to be severely deficient, even early in HIV infection. Researchers at the University of Miami have recommended PWHIV supplement with a minimum of 75 mg. per day. Please check zinc sources in any other multivitamin and antioxidant complexes before adding additional zinc to a protocol. Zinc has been helpful in correcting problems of taste and smell as well as helping with various skin disorders.

A critical nutrient in the immune response, zinc has been shown to increase natural killer cells, cell mediated immunity and phagocytosis (the ingestion of foreign or damaged material by immune cells). Zinc also strengthens macrophages and is essential for the health of the thymus gland and lymph nodes. Several recent studies with PWHIVs have documented the immune stimulatory qualities of zinc.

For optimal absorption, zinc should be taken with vitamins B-6 and A. Daily zinc should not exceed 50 mg. if there is a candida albicans or bacterial infection. Zinc in excess of 150 mg per day may decrease phagocytic activity, neutrophils and macrophages.

Copper is another deficient trace mineral in HIV infection. Researchers have recorded that 74 percent of PWHIVs have a copper deficiency. Common signs of a copper deficiency are heart flutters or palpitations. Copper is necessary for antibody response, infection resistance and cell mediated immunity. Check all sources of copper from multivitamin and antioxidant complexes before adding additional copper. Because they compete for absorption, copper and zinc should not be taken at the same time.

Amino Acids

Amino acids should be taken on an empty stomach 20 minutes before or 90 minutes after eating.

Amino acids promote human protein production. In HIV infection, they need to be resupplied in order to promote cell functioning and depletion from HIV infection.

Carnitine

Several reports indicate the systemic carnitine deficiency could occur in AIDS, and that primary and secondary carnitine deficiency leads to critical metabolic dysfunctions. In a significant Italian study of 28 PWHIVs, 6 grams of carnitine was administered for just two weeks. Immune responsiveness was greatly enhanced as well as significant reductions in Beta-2 microglobulin. More importantly, Tumor Necrosis Factor (TNF) levels were normalized in the two study participants who had abnormally high levels, while triglyceride levels were reduced on average approximately 35 percent. Triglycerides levels are a secondary marker for high TNF levels in the body. High TNF levels has been implicated as a central immune dysregulation, which can greatly foster disease through the mechanism of early cell death (apoptosis), since TNF produces large quantities of free radicals.

Glutathione (GSH)

Resupplying GSH in HIV/AIDS is essential for restoring vital vitamin C and E antioxidant action. It protects cells/organs against broad range oxidative damage and other toxicities. It can slow or stop chronic intracellular viral activations and restore cellular immune responsiveness as well as perform many other critical immune functions. This global sulfur (thiol) deficiency potentiates HIV replication and accelerates disease progression.

Adequate levels of GSH are required for mixed lymphocyte reactions, T-cell proliferation, T and B cell differentiation, cytotoxic T-cell activity, and natural killer cell activity. Drugs that replenish GSH counteract oxidative stress and inhibit HIV transcription and replication in models of acute and latent HIV infection.

Dr. Wolf Droge, one of the researchers who discovered the GSH deficiency in 1989, has just released a research report stating that AIDS is possibly the result of a viral induced cysteine deficiency. He makes this statement after reviewing the GSH levels in several primate (monkey) models who do not proceed to immune suppression after being infected with HIV. He discovered that these monkeys, unlike humans, never lose the substantial amounts of GSH and other thiols within their blood or their cells.

The loss of this critical group of sulfur amino acids, mainly cysteine, which is the building block used in the manufacture of GSH, alters host defense to such a degree as to account for all further disease progression.

Because of the high amino acid glutamate levels in HIV infection, various forms of cysteine are actually blocked from being used by immune cells. Therefore, a mixture of different sulfur amino acids (thiols) and GSH itself is thought to be the wisest course of action in replacing glutathione.

Research has shown that as HIV disease increases, cellular levels of GSH decrease. Since research has demonstrated that GSH is critical to the immune response and to the prevention of premature apoptosis (self-destruction of impaired cells whose membranes have become leaky and lost sufficient GSH, which controls the cell cycle), then resupplying cysteine, the major component of GSH, is absolutely critical.

Glutathione has also been shown in laboratory conditions to either dramatically reduce active viruses, including HIV and herpes viruses, or to stop the reactivation of latent virus inside cells.

Researchers recommend taking sulfur amino acids in a multifactorial mixture. This is because GSH is composed of three amino acids is most bioavailable in this form. GSH also should be taken along with methionine and albumin. Methionine stops the breakdown of GSH by the liver in an attempt to retrieve the cysteine portion of the molecule and albumin is a protein transporter for GSH.

N-Acetyl-L-Cysteine (NAC)

N-Acetyl-L-Cysteine (NAC) is an amino acid derivative of L-cysteine and a precursor of GSH.

In a Pasteur Institute study, NAC stopped premature apoptosis, one of the leading models for immune cell loss. NIH laboratory studies have also demonstrated that NAC is effective as and antioxidant, increases GSH and has antiviral activity, all of which is critical in the treatment of HIV infection.

NAC should be taken at at least 2,000 mg. per day, preferably on an empty stomach 20 minutes before or 90 minutes after eating. NAC is quite acidic and may, if taken along with vitamin C, cause stomach upset. If this occurs, NAC can be taken along with food or with betaine hydrochloride.

Botanical Substances

DAAIR currently is extremely conservative in using herbal combinations. Many herbs traditionally used to fight viral illnesses and chronic infection can actually increase these dysfunctional hyper-abnormal immune productions. A good example of this is the herb echinacae, which is now known to increase TNF, which generates excess free radicals and can increase viral replication.

However, there are some botanical substances that can be recommended.

Artemesia

This has been found to be very useful for treating parasites.

Astragalus

This herb is an adaptogen. It tends to normalize abnormal, stressed physiology. A primary problem in HIV infection is inflammatory immune dysregulation with the accompanying overproduction of certain key inflammatory immune messengers (cytokines) and increased free radical generation. Astragalus also has been proven clinically useful in raising white blood cell counts when used in combination with chemotherapy.

Bioflavonoids (Including Quercitin)

Bioflavonoids have been shown to increase the effectiveness of vitamin C. Quercitin is a bioflavonoid derived from blue-green algae and an antioxidant and antihistamine that has been shown to have antiviral activity. In addition, it is synergistic with vitamin C.

Bioflavonoids are potent protectors of free-radical damage in plants and are part of a multifactorial approach to controlling the inflammatory immune over-activation found in HIV disease

Chlorella and Alfalfa

Chlorella is a whole food product and therefore contains many factors not found in isolates, including over 12 pigments, which are the precursors of enzymes and co-enzymes. This is a good product to use when a diet does not contain high amounts of green leafy vegetables.

Garlic

High dose garlic (between 5 and 7.5 grams per day) is a central component of the DAAIR protocol and is suggested for anyone who is interested in a broad range anti-bacterial/fungal/viral with proven clinical ability to improve immune function. In several small studies, it increased T-4 cell numbers, improved T-4 / T8 ratios and normalized low natural killer cell activity. Partial symptom resolution was also reported (e.g., cryptosporidia diarrhea, recurring genital herpes and aggressive candidiasis).

Garlic is being intensively studied for its many potent biological qualities. Garlic extracts inhibit many microbes that commonly cause opportunistic infections in AIDS, including cytomegalovirus, herpes simplex 1 and 2, staph, salmonella, parasites, TB, entamoeba, histoplasmosis and mycobacterium avium.

Ginkgo Biloba

Some PWHIVs believe Gingko extracts may be helpful in providing antioxidant action, reducing chronic inflammation (particularly of the central and peripheral nervous systems, which HIV definitely attacks), enhancing oxygen supply and improving cerebral (brain) functions of memory and retention.

Ginseng (Siberian)

This adaptogen restores altered physiology toward normal. It contains trace minerals, vitamins and oils. Thirty years of Russian research revealed that Siberian Ginseng exerts a balancing effect, helping to correct either an excess or deficiency in the body, like astragalus. DAAIR recommends alternation Siberian ginseng once a month with astragalus.

Glycyrrhizin (GL)

This highly refined extract of licorice can be purchased from DAAIR in prescription and non-prescription formulas. GL is a potent antiviral and anti-inflammatory. It has offered PWAs and some PWHIVs full clinical stabilization with immune restoration/normalization under some clinical circumstances.

Milk Thistle

This is a potent liver-strengthening compound. It stimulates the liver to regenerate itself by producing new liver cells as well as having strong antioxidant action to help prevent lipid-peroxidation of cell membranes. Given to 7 patients receiving tuberculosis drugs (INH and ethambutol), a standardized silymarin extract normalized elevated liver enzymes after 3 months treatment.

Recently, Chilean researchers have discovered that silymarin increases glutathione in the liver, stomach and intestines by over 50 percent, although it did not increase GSH levels in other organs.

Tumeric

Tumeric has been used in Aurveydic (Indian) medicine for several thousand years. The extract from the herb tumeric is known to be a potent anti-inflammatory and antioxidant.

In laboratory work at Harvard University, it was shown to be an effective inhibitor of viral incorporation into cells, as well as an inhibitor of viral activity in chronically infected cells (virus that has already been incorporated into cells and is actively replicating).

Anecdotal evidence in small numbers of PWHIVs has shown reductions in P24 antigen activity (the viral protein release into the blood) as well as reductions in the inflammatory marker Beta-2-Microglobulin.

Other Special Substances

Bifidus and Lactic Acid producing Bacteria

These products are considered essential, due to the malabsorption and GI tract immune dysfunction found early in HIV infection

Bifidus is a friendly micro-organism that may be the first organism to appear in the healthy intestinal tract. it has been found in large quantities in newborn babies. Research has shown that L. Bifidus inhibits the growth of common disease-causing bacteria, including coliforms, salmonella and candida. It also works with L. acidophilus to benefit digestion and the production of B vitamins.

L. acidophilus supports immune functions that promote resistance to infections, which may in turn enhance immunity to certain diseases. It has been shown to fight off and displace undesirable and potentially destructive bacteria and yeast in the gastrointestinal tract. These L. acidophilus organisms facilitate the digestibility of protein, help to produce B vitamins, enhance calcium absorption and stimulate enzymatic activities involved with absorption of nutrients.

Essential Fatty Acids

Essential Fatty Acids (EFAs) are deficient even at early stages of HIV infection. They are incorporated into the cell membranes and greatly help to reduce inflammatory by-products that are over-produced in the HIV dysfunctional immune response. Used clinically for many varied skin problems in HIV disease, EFAs are long-term, anti-inflammatories that also may help with fatigue and loss of sense of smell and taste.

Thioctic Acid

Research in Germany suggests that this potent antioxidant and liver protective agent is even stronger as an antioxicant than NAC. At the same time, it has proven capabilities to protect many organs and tissues from free radicals.

In laboratory conditions, thioctic acid has been shown to be a more potent inhibitor of the activation of latent HIV (still dormant within cells) than NAC.

This is an indispensable agent for anyone who uses long-term, liver-toxic, prophylactic drugs, or to provide further protection from other kinds of liver damage. It also is excellent for those with impaired liver functions who want to take high dose garlic. Another broad-spectrum antioxidant, thioctic acid should be a part of the protocol of any PWHIV who is interested in the most extensive multifactorial mix of free radical protecting agents.

PWHIVs should let their doctor know that they are taking this compound. It will allow them to tolerate much higher doses of liver-toxic drugs than would normally be the case. Thioctic acid never should be stopped suddenly while continuing to take pharmaceutical agents without closely monitoring liver enzyme levels.

Section III

Resources

Notes from A Long-Term Survivor

When Dr. Goh asked me to write this piece as a long-term survivor, it set into motion a cascade of thoughts and memories. As someone who was infected before we knew AIDS existed, I immediately realized that my point of view is shaped by a time when I had to take charge of my own treatment or die.

In a sense, this is still true today. In the end, it is I who must make the final decision in any medical matter. This attitude has saved my life several times. Since 1983, when I had to confront that horrifying fact of survival, I have been able to create and develop my own eclectic treatment regimen. This regimen includes several health modalities: Western medicine, acupuncture, Chiropractic, herbs, shiatsu and therapeutic massage.

Many might think that these treatments are beyond the financial reach of people like me, who is on disability. However, I am living proof that this is not so. I could write a whole book about the many financial problems that are related to obtaining HIV and AIDS treatment regimens, and all of the health and medical disasters that can occur because of those financial problems. Instead, I want to list briefly those treatments that have worked for me.

The first treatment tool available to me in the early eighties was Chiropractic adjustments. Contrary to popular belief, Chiropractic is not just a "bone doctor" treatment. It is a complex interrelationship between the vertebra of the body and the nervous system. Like a garden hose that has been stepped on, an incorrect vertebrae can weaken the body's ability to work properly with the nervous system.

The second treatment tool that I was able to utilize was visualization. Visualization is indispensable for programming my brain to live with this infection and survive. Even Einstein felt that he only used 10 percent of his brain. The immune system in our bodies uses lymphocytes, antigens and other cellular defenses. The brain's ability to focus, harness and direct the body's immune defense system can be greatly expanded through visualization.

Acupuncture and herbs were added to my treatment regimen at around the same time. They created remarkable changes in my health, as well as a major change in the way I view treatment. Like most everyone else infected with HIV, I was attempting to kill the virus, preferably with a "Magic Bullet." However, through my acupuncturists and herbalists, I discovered that every time we try to kill a virus in the body, we kill or hurt the body as well.

The other concept I learned was that the human body has been able to live with innumerable viruses.

Therefore, the goal for me in alternative HIV treatments is to try to teach my body to live with the virus.

With this understanding, I would like to explain what has worked for me, a long-term survivor, who has outlived the CDC's own projections of HIV disease progression many times over. Besides avoiding AZT and its many evil analogs, my treatment plan includes five major supporting modalities:

1. Herbs

Herb Tea #1 has been vitally important, not only in keeping many blood markers within normal range, but also in maintaining a quality of life that is acceptable to me and superior to most of my contemporaries. I also must mention its beneficial, long-term effect on my damaged liver. I have gone from being refused from studies due to high liver enzymes to an almost perfectly normal liver panel. The potential for Herb Tea #1 as a buffer drug should not be overlooked, since many treatments are very hard on the liver. As a person who is allergic or sensitive to many drugs, I find its lack of side-effects very pleasing.

2. Acupuncture

Acupuncture is a most amazing tool after you get over the idea of having needles stuck into your body. The discomfort has been greatly exaggerated. I can actually be put to sleep with needles. Acupuncture also can help other medications to become more effective and reduce their side-effects. These side-effects alone, which often can result in a major hospitalization, can be cleared up with out-patient acupuncture treatments.

Acupuncture can begin to show dramatic results with as few as five treatments. However, like any treatment regimen, acupuncture must be done regularly over a long period of time for its full potential to be realized. I have received from one to three treatments per week over the past five years.

3. Chiropractic

Chiropractic is another amazing tool because of its obvious immune boosting benefits to a freely flowing nervous system. Chiropractic is a veritable treasure of preventative techniques. Like acupuncture, this treatment requires regular application in order to optimize the benefits. I have been under Chiropractic care for 12 years.

4. Shiatsu and Therapeutic Massage

Shiatsu is similar to acupuncture, but without needles. Again, it unblocks or balances the body's energy flow. But, it also can be a valuable diagnostic tool. Therapeutic massage also is essential, not only to keep range of motion as free as possible, but also to experience the healing contact of human touch. This physical contact is essential to people who have become physically or emotionally isolated by illness.

5. Medical

"Diagnosis and treatment by consensus" is the only way to become empowered. It is imperative to find an MD who will work with you rather than dictate to you. Some people dismiss doctors because they have failed to produce a "cure." This is risky. There are few things as useful as a caring physician. He or she can help you to monitor your well-being. Medical tests, blood work and opinions are important in helping to judge whether something is healing or hurting. But, how you feel about the particular treatment is essential to the future decisions you will have to make about your health. Consultations with a doctor that you trust is important in helping you to create and maintain a treatment approach that is designed by you and that works for you.

6. Nutrition

Last but not least is the fuel that you put into your body. What special vitamins and nutrients you may decide to take should be based not only on blood work but on how the food or substance makes you feel.

When utilizing "food therapy," simply relying on blood tests is a mistake. Depending on which physical problems exist, some foods or supplements may not be right. For example, liver and ulcer problems may limit foods that might be helpful for HIV. The problem of following pre-set diets is that they can cancel out other possible beneficial effects. Ask yourself how your body is reacting to a given nutrient or food. Ask yourself how it makes you feel. There is no point in taking something that makes you feel badly the next day.

In Summary...

Because of the early intervention I have taken in using alternative treatments for HIV infection, I have lived longer than I ever dreamed possible. I have also lived better. And, as a long-term survivor, I am not able to be picked out in a crowd as a Person Living With AIDS.

Michael D. Anderson

Finding Alternative Treatments

Pages 230-236 of this listing includes a range of professional associations that can assist in the reader in locating alternative treatment practitioners across the country. This listing was provided by the Office of Alternative Medicine, the National Institutes of Health. These associations are grouped by type of alternative or complementary medical treatment approach. Their inclusion in this list does not constitute endorsement of any of the associations by the Office of Alternative Medicine.

Page 237 includes a short listing of organizations or clinics that either were mentioned in the book or that provide more direct information or alternative treatments for HIV/AIDS.

Pages 238-246 includes a state listing of AIDS organizations. This listing was printed by permission of Gay Men's Health Crisis, New York City, from their guide, entitled, *Living with AIDS.*

Holistic Health Care

Alliance for Alternatives in Healthcare
PO Box 9178
Calabasas, CA 913 72
(818) 702-0888
Holistic Medicine
Steve Gorman, President

Alliance / Foundation for Alternative Medicine
160 NW Widmer Place
Albany, OR 97321

American Foundation for Alternative Healthcare, Research and Development
25 Landfield Avenue
Monticello, NY 12701
(914) 794-8181
Holistic Medicine
Edwin M. Field, Executive Dir.

American Association of Naturopathic Physicians
PO Box 20386
Seattle, WA 98102
(206) 323-7610

American Holistic Medical Association
4101 Lake Boon Trail
Suite 201
Raleigh, NC 27607
(919) 787-5181

American Holistic Nurses Association
4101 Lake Boone Trail
Suite 201
Raleigh, NC 27607
(919) 787-5181
Cathy Young, Exec. Dir.

American Holistic Veterinary Medical Association
2214 Old Emmorton Road
Bel Air, MD 21015
(410) 569-0795

Committee for Freedom of Choice in Medicine
1180 Walnut Avenue
Chula Vista, CA 92011
(800) 227-4473

Holistic Dental Association
974 North 21st Street
Newark, OH 43055
(614) 366-3309

International Association of Holistic Health Practitioners
3419 Thom Boulevard
Las Vegas, NV 89130
((702) 873-4542
Dr. Joseph Kadams, Exec. Dir.

Mankind Research Foundation
1315 Apple Avenue
Silver Spring, MD 20910
(301) 587-8686
Holistic Health
Dr. Carl Schleicher, Pres.

Nurses in Transition
PO Box 104
Genco, CA 95232
Holistic Health
Diane Dichesae, Exec. Dir.

Serendipity Association for Research and Implementation of Holistic Health and World Peace
3970 Florida Street, #AG09
San Diego, CA 92104
(619) 297-8902

Diet / Nutrition / Lifestyle Changes

American Natural Hygiene Society
11816 Racetrack Road
Tampa, FL 33626
(813) 855-6607

International Association of Professional Natural Hygienists
204 Stambaugh Building
Youngstown, OH 44503
(813) 855-6607

Physicians Committee for Responsible Medicine
PO Box 6322
Washington, DC 20015
(202) 686-2210

Mind / Body Control Interventions

Aloha International
PO Box 665
Kilauea, HI 96754
(800) 877-7277
Huna Therapy, Shaman Training
Serge King, Ph.D., Exec. Director

American Association for Therapeutic Humoor
12 South Hanley Street
St. Louis, MO 63105
(305) 948-3010

Anthroposophical Nurses Association of America
Rural Route #2
Box 210
Ghent, NY 12075

Association for Humanistic Psychology
1772 Vallejo Street
San Francisco, CA 94123
(415) 346-7929

Association for Past-Life Research and Therapies
PO Box 20151
Riverside, CA 92516
(714) 784-1570

Consciousness Research and Training Project
315 East 68th Street, Box 9G
New York, NY 10021
Parapsychology, Meditation, Healing
Joyce Goodrich, Ph.D., President

Himalayan International Institute of Yoga Science and Philosophy of the USA
RR #1, Box 400
Honesdale, PA 18431
(717) 253-5551
Yoga / Meditation, Holistic Health
Rudolph M. Ballantine, MD, President

International Society for the Study of Subtle Energies and-Energy Medicine (ISSSSEEM)
356 Goldco Circle
Golden, CO 80401
(303) 278-2228

Physicians Association for Anthroposophical Medicine
PO Box 269
Kimberton, PA 19442

Hypnotherapy

Academy of Scientific Hypnotherapy
PO Box 12041
San Diego, CA 92112
(619) 427-6225

American Association of Professional Hypnotherapists
PO Box 29
Boones Mill, VA 24065
(703) 334-3035

American Council of Hypnotist Examiners
312 Riverdale Drive
Glendale, CA 91204
(818) 242-1159

American Society of Clinical Hypnosis
2200 East Devon, Suite 291
Des Plaines, IL 60018
(708) 297-3317

International Medical and Dental Hypnotherapy Association
4110 Edgeland, Suite 800
Royal Oak, MI 48073
(313) 549-5594

National Society of Hypnotherapists
2175 NW 86th, Suite 6A
Des Moines, IA 50325
(515) 270-2280

Art / Music / Dance Therapy

American Art Therapy Association, Incorporated
1202 Allanson Road
Mundelein, IL 60060
(708) 949-6064

American Dance Therapy Association
2000 Century Plaza, Suite 108
Columbia, MD 21044
(410) 997-4040

Dinshah Health Society
100 Dinshah Drive
Malaga, NJ 08328
(609) 692-4684
Color / Light Therapy
Danus Dinshah, President

National Association for Music Therapy
8455 Colesville Road, Suite 930
Silver Spring, MD 20910
(301) 589-3300

Radiance Technique Association International
PO Box 40570
St. Petersberg, FL 33743
(813) 347-3421
Radiance Therapy
Fred W. Wright, Executive Director

Acupuncture and Traditional Chinese Medicine

Acupuncture International Association
2330 South Brentwood Boulevard
St. Louis, MO 63144
(314) 961-2300
Dr. Carol Ann Lee, Vice President

Acupuncture Research Institute
313 West Andrix Street
Monterey Park, CA 91754
(213) 722-7353
Acupuncture, Homeopathy
Louis Gasper, Ph.D., Executive Secretary

American Academy of Medical Acupuncture
5820 Wilshire Boulevard, Suite 500
Los Angeles, CA 90036
(213) 937-5514

American Acupuncture Association
4262 Kissena Boulevard
Flushing, NY 11355
(718) 886-4431

American Association of Acupuncture and Oriental Medicine
1400 16th Street, NW, Suite 710
Washington, DC 20036
(202) 265-2287
Acupuncture, Oriental Medicine
Yvette Williams, National Office Director

American Foundation of Traditional Chinese Medicine
1280 Columbus Avenue, Suite 302
San Francisco, CA 94133
(415) 776-0502
Oriental Healing, Acupuncture
Barbara Bernie, President

American Oriental Bodywork Therapy Association
50 Maple Place
Manhattan, NY 11030
(516) 365-5025

East West Academy of Healing Arts
450 Sutter, Suite 916
San Francisco, CA 94108
(415) 788-2227
Qigong, Oriental Medicine
Dr. Effie Chow, President

International Foundation of Oriental Medicine
PO Box 625
Oakland Gardens, NY 11364
(718) 321-8642

International Veterinary Acupuncture Society
2140 Conestoga Road
Chester Springs, PA 19425
(215) 827-7245

Maharishi Ayurveda Association of America
PO Box 282
Fairfield, IA 52556
(515) 472-8477

Homeopathy

Homeopathic Academy of Naturopathic Physicians
14653 South Graves Road
Mulino, OR 97042
(503) 829-7326

Homeopathic Council for Research and Education
50 Park Avenue
New York, NY 10016
Dr. William Bergman, MD

International Foundation for Homeopathy
2366 Eastlake Avenue East, #30
Seattle, WA 98102
(206) 324-8230
Homeopathic Medicine
Fred Bishop, Executive Director

National Center for Homeopathy
801 North Fairfax Streeet, Suite 306
Alexandria, VA 22314
(708) 548-7790

Herbalism

Alternative Medicine Association
7907 SE Stark Street
Portland, OR 97215

American Herbalists Build
PO Box 1863
Soquel, CA 95073
(408) 438-1700

American Herb Association
PO Box 1673
Nevada City, CA 95959
(916) 265-9552

Structural and Energetic Therapies

American Healing Association
c/o Rev. Brian Zink
811 Ridge Drive
Glendale, CA 91206
healing

Touch for Health Foundation
1174 North Lake Avenue
Pasadena, CA 91104
(818) 794-1181
Touch Therapy, Holistic Health, Library of 500+ Volumes
Forrest Turpen, Executive Director

North American Academy of Musculoskeletal Medicine
7611 Elmwood Avenue, Suite 202
Middleton, WI 33562
(608) 831-9240
Manual Manipulation
Barbara Johns, Executive Director

Chiropractic

American Chiropractic Assiciation
1701 Clarendon Boulevard
Arlington, VA 22209
(202) 276-8800
J. Ray Morgan, Executive Vice President

Association of Chiropractic Colleges
2005 Via Barrett, Box 367
San Lorenzo, CA 94580
(510) 276-9013
Gerald W. Clum, DC, President
Clearinghouse of Chiropractic and Holistic Health Information

Association for History of Chiropractic
c/o Encyclopedia of Associations
835 Penobscot Building
Detroit, MI 48226

Association for Network Chiropractic
3075 Emmons Avenue
Brooklyn, NY 11235
(718) 891-4077

Flying Chiropractors Association
7301 Hasbrook Avenue
Philadelphia, PA 19111
(215) 722-7200
Dr. W.J. Quinlin, Executive Director

Foundation for Chiropractic Education and Research
1701 Clarendon Boulevarde
Arlington, VA 22209
(703) 276-7445
Steve Seater, CAE, Executive Director

International Chirpractors Association (ICA)
1110 North Glebe Road, Suite 1000
Arlington, VA 22201
(703) 528-5000

National Directory of Chiropractic
PO Box 10056
Olathe, KS 66051
(800) 888-7914

Sacro Occipital Research Society International
PO Box 8245
Prairie Billage, KS 66208
(913) 384-2784
Cranial Osteopathy, Chiropractic
Dr. Cameron DeCamp, President

World Chiropractic Alliance
2950 North Dobson Road, Suite 1
Chandler, AZ 85224
(800) 347-1011

Massage / Bodywork

American Alliance of Massage Professionals
3108 Route 10 West
Denville, NJ 07834
(201) 989-8941

American Massage Therapy Association
1130 West North Shore Avenue
Chicago, IL 60626
(312) 761- AMTA

American Polarity Therapy Association
4101 Lake Boone Trail
Raleigh, NC 27607
(919) 787-5181

Asociated Bodywork and Massage Professionals
PO Box 489
Evergreen, CO 80439
(303) 647-8478
(800) 8-MASSAGE

Feldenkrais Guild
524 Ellsworth Street
PO Box 489
Albany, OR 97321
(503) 926-0981

Foot Reflexology Awareness Association
PO Box 7622
Mission Hills, CA 91346
(818) 361-0528

International Association of Infant-Massage Instruction (IAIMI)
2350 Bowen Road, PO Box 438
Elmira, NY 14059
(716) 652-9789

International College of Applied Kinesiology
PO Box 905
Lawrence, KS 66044
(913) 542-1801
Acupressure, Touch and Massage Therapy

International Rolf Institute
302 Pearl Street
Boulder, CO 80306
(303) 449-5903

North American Society of Teachers of the Alexander Technique
PO Box 3992
Champaign, IL 61826
(217) 359-3529

Nurse Healers Association
234 Fifth Avenue, #3399
New York, NY 10001
(518) 325-3583

Reiki Alliance
PO Box 41
Cataldo, ID 83810
(208) 682-3535

Touch for Health Association
7159 Manchester Avenue
Maplewood, MO 63143
(800) 466-TFHA

Chelation

American Board of Chelation Therapy
70 West Huron Street
Chicago, IL 60610
(312) 787-ABCT

American College of Advancement in Medicin
23121 Verdugo Drive, Suite 204
Laguna Hills, CA 92653
(714) 583-7666
(800) LEAD-OUT

Aromatherapy

Aromatherapy Institute of Research
PO Box 2354
Fair Oaks, CA 95628
(916) 965-7546

Flower Essence Society
PO Box 459
Nevada City, CA 95959
(916) 265-9163

National Association of Holistic Aromatherapists
PO Box 17622
Boulder, CO 80308
(303)447-9598
(303) 258-3792

Vision Therapy

American Optometric Association (AOA)
243 North Lindbergh Boulevard
St. Louis, MO 63141
(314) 991-4100

College of Optometrists and Vision Development
PO Box 385
Chula Vista, CA 91912
(619) 425-6191

Optometric Extension Program Foundation, Incorporated (OEP)
2912 Daimler Street
Santa Ana, CA 92705
(714) 250-8070

Other Alternative Approaches

Alzheimer's Association
919 North Michigan Avenue, Suite 1000
Chicago, IL 60611
(800) 272-3900
Alternative Alzheimer's Therapies

American Academy of Environmental Medicin
PO Box 16106
Denver, CO 80216
(303) 622-9755
Alternative Alergy Therapies

International Association for Oxigen Therapy
PO Box 1360
Priest River, ID 83856
(208) 448-2504

National Iridology research Association
PO Box 1278
Glenneyre, #153
Laguna Beach, CA 92651

Cancer

Arlin J. Brown Information Center
PO Box 251
Fort Belvoir, CA 22060
(707) 752-9511
Information on Non-Toxic Cancer Therapies

Cancer Control Society
2304 North Berendo Street
Los Angeles, CA 90027
(213) 663-7801
Information on Cancer Clinics

CanHelp
3111 Paradise Bay Road
Port Ludlow, WA 98365-9771
(206) 437-2291
Information on Alternative Cancer Therapies

Foundation for Advancement in Cancer Therapy (FACT)
PO Box 1242 Old Chelsea Station
New York, NY 10113
(212) 741-2790
also:
PO Box 215
200 East Lancaster Avenue
Wynnwood, PA 19096
(215) 642-4810
Information on Non-Toxic Therapies

Health Resource
209 Katherine Drive
Conway, AK 72032
(501) 329-8700
Individualized Cancer Research Reports

People Against Cancer
PO Box 10
Otho, IA 50569-0010
(515) 972-4444
FAX: (515) 972-4415
Information on Alternative and Conventional Cancer Therapies

HIV/AIDS Alternative Treatments

AIDS Care Project
140 Clarenden Street
Boston, MA 02116
(617) 859-3026

Austin Immune Health Clinic, Incorporated
5605 Bennett Avenue
Austin, TX 78741
(512) 327-2883

Heatlh Education AIDS Liaison (HEAL)
PO Box 1103
Old Chelsea Station
New York, NY 10113
(800) 410-HEAL
Michael Ellner, President

Immune Enhancement Project
3450 16th Street
San Francisco, CA 94114
(415) 252-8711

Kang Wen Clinic
1111 Harvard Hill
1 Baptist Church
Seattle, WA 98122
(206) 233-8936

Lincoln Medical and Mental Health Center
Acupuncture Clinic
349 East 140th Street
Bronx, NY 10454
(212) 993-3100
Michael O. Smith, MD

Magnolia Health Center
383 Fifth Avenue, 4th Floor
New York, NY 10016
(212) 213-0118
Dr. Magnolia Goh

Portland Acupuncture Addiction Center
1201 SW Morrison
Portland, OR 97205
(503) 228-4533

Quan Yin Healing Arts Center
1748 Market Street
San Francisco, CA 94102
(415) 861-1101

Treatment Education Program
AIDS Project Los Angeles
1313 North Vine Street
Los Angeles, CA 90028
(213) 993-1482

Alabamba

AIDS Task Force of Alabama
PO Box 55703
Birmingham, AL 35255
(205) 324-2437

Alaska

Alaskan AIDS Assistance Association
730 I Street, #100
Anchorage, AK 99501
(907) 276-4480
(800) 478-AIDS (In-state only)

Arizona

Tuscon AIDS Project
151 South Tuscon Boulevard, Suite 252
Tuscon, AZ 85716
(602) 322-6226

Arkansas

Arkansas AIDS Project
5911 H Street
Little Rock, AR 72205
(501) 663-7833

California

AIDS Project Los Angeles (APLA)
1313 North Vine Street
Los Angeles, CA 90028
(800) 922-2437 Hotline
(213) 962-1600 Office
(800) 922-2438 Multi-languagel line
(800) 533-2437 TDD line

San Francisco AIDS Foundation
25 Van Ness Avenue, Suite 660
San Francisco, CA 94142
(415) 863-AIDS San Francisco Hotline
(800) FOR-AIDS Toll free in Northern California
(415) 864-6606 TDD line

Shanti Project
Laguna Beach, CA 92651
(714) 949-1446

Shanti Project
6855 Santa Monica Boulevard, #405
Los Angeles, CA 90028
(213) 962-8197

Shanti Project
525 Howard Street
San Francisco, CA 94105
(415) 777-2273

Colorado

Boulder County AIDS Project
2188 14th Street
Boulder, CO 80302
(303) 444-6121

Colorado AIDS Project (CAP)
Box 18529, 1576 Sherman
Denver, CO 80203
(303) 837-0166

Gay & Lesbian Community Center of Colorado
PO Drawer E
Denver, CO 80218
(303) 831-6268

Connecticut

AIDS Project Hartford
30 Arbor Street
Hartford, CT 06106-1209
(203) 247-2437

AIDS Project New Haven
PO Box 636
New Haven, CT 06503
(203) 624-0947
(203) 624-AIDS Hotline 6:30-9:30 p.m.

Delaware

AIDS Program Office
Division of Public Health, Building G
Wilmington, DE 19808
(800) 422-0429

Delaware Lesbian/Gay Health Advocates
800 West Street
Wilmington, DE 19801
(302) 652-6776

District of Columbia

National Lesbian & Gay Health Foundation
1407 S Street, NW
Washington, DC 20009
(202) 797-3578

National Association of People with AIDS (NAPWA)
1413 K Street, NW, 8th Floor
Washington, DC 20006
(202) 898-0414

Whitman-Walker Clinic
1407 S Street, NW
Washington, DC 20009
(202) 332-AIDS Hotline
(202) 332-5295 Client Services

Florida

Florica AIDS/HIV Hotline
PO Box 20169
Tallahassee, FL 32316
(800) FLA-AIDS
(800) 545-SIDA (Spanish)
(800) AIDS-101 (Hatian/Creole)

Miami AIDS Project
University of Miami School of Medicine
1800 NW Tenth Avenue, 1st Floor
Miami, FL 33163
(305) 547-3838

Georgia

AID-Atlanta
1132 West Peachtree Street, NW
Atlanta, GA 30309
(404) 872-0600 Client Services
(404) 876-9944 Infoline
(800) 551-2728 Infoline (In-state only)

Hawaii

Life Foundation
PO Box 88980
Honolulu, HI 96830
(808) 971-2437

Idaho

Idaho AIDS Foundation
PO Box 421
Boise, ID 83701-4321
(208) 345-2277
(800) 677-2437 Infoline

Illinois

AIDS Foundation Chicago
1332 North Halstead, #303
Chicago, IL 60622
(312) 642-5454
(312) 642-3763 Hotline

Howard Brown Health Center
945 West George Street
Chicago, IL 60657
(312) 871-5777

Horizons Community Services
961 West Montana
Chicago, IL 60614
(312) 472-6494
(800) 243-2437 (In-state only)
(800) 782-1423 TDD

Indiana

Indiana AIDS Hotline
(800) 848-2437

Damien Center
1350 North Pennsylvania
Indianapolis, IN 46202
(317) 632-0123

Indiana Community AIDS Action Network (ICAAN)
3951 North Meridian, Suite 200
Indianapolis, IN 46208
(307) 920-3190
(800) 659-7850 Helpline

Iowa

Iowa Department of Public Health
AIDS Prevention Program
Lucas Building, 1st Floor
Des Moines, IA 50319
(515) 281-6801
(800) 445-2437 (In-state only)

Kansas

Topeka AIDS Project
1615 West 8th Street
PO Box 4726
Topeka, KS 66604-4726
(913) 232-3100 AIDS Project

Kentucky

AIDS Volunteer
214 West Maxwell Street
Lexington, KY 40585
PO Box 431
Lexington, KY 40585-0431
(606) 254-2865

Louisiana

New Orleans AIDS Task Force
1407 Decatur Street
New Orleans, LA 70116
(504) 945-4000 Office
(504) 944-2437 Hotline
(800) 992-4379 Hotline

Maine

The AIDS Project
22 Monument Squre, 5th Floor
Portland, ME 04101
(207) 775-1267
(207) 774-6877 Hotline
(800) 851-AIDS Hotline (In-state only)

Maryland

Health Education Resource Organization (HERO)
101 West Reade Street, Suite 825
Baltimore, MD 21201
(410) 945-AIDS Hotline
(410) 685-1180 Client Services

Massachusetts

AIDS Action Committee
131 Clarendon Street
Boston, MA 02116
(617) 437-6200
(617) 437 1394 TDD

Massachusetts Hotlines
(800) 235-2331 (In-state only)
(617) 536-7733 Hotline
(800) 788-1234 Youth Hotline
(617) 437-1672 TDD

Michigan

The AIDS Project
Detroit Heatlh Department
1151 Taylor
Detroit, MI 48202
(313) 876-0980

Minnesota

Minnesota AIDS Project
2025 Nicollet Avenue, Suite 200
Minneapolis, MN 55404
(612) 870-7773
(612) 870-0700 Metro AIDS line
(800) 248-2437 (In-state only)

Mississippi

Mississippi HIV Education and Prevention Program
Mississippi State Board of Health
2423 North State Street, Box 1700
Jackson, MS 39215-1700
(601) 960-7723
(800) 826-2961 Hotline

Missouri

Good Samaritan AIDS Project
3030 Walnut Street
Kansas City, MO 64108
(816) 561-8780
(800) 5 6 1-8780 Hotline

Montana

Yellowstone AIDS Project
3030 Second Avenue North
Billings, MT 590-101
(406) 245-2029
(800)675-2437 (In-state only)

Nebraska

Nebraska AIDS Project
3624 Leavenworth Street
Omaha, NE 68105
(402) 342-6367
(800) 782-2437 Hotline

Nevada

Aid for AIDS of Nevada (AFAN)
1111 Desert Lane
Las Vegas, NV 89102
(702) 382-2326
(702) 474-2437 Hotline

Nevada State Health Division
505 East King Street, Room 304
Carson City, NV 89710
(702) 687-4800
(702) 842-2437 Infoline

New Hampshire

New Hampshire AIDS Foundation
PO Box 59
Manchester, NH 03105-0059
(603) 623-0710
(800) 639-1122 Infoline

New Hampshire Department of Health
Health and Welfare Building
6 Hazen Drive
Concord, NH 03301
(603) 271-4502
(800) 752-2437 Hotline (In-state only)

New Jersey

Hyacinth AIDS Foundation
103 Bayard Street
New Brunswick, NJ 08901
(800) 433-0254 Hotline (In-state only)
(908) 246-0204

New Jersey AIDS Hotline
(800) 624-2377
(201) 926-8008 TDD

New Mexico

New Mexico AIDS Services
4200 Silver Street, SE, Suite B
Albuquerque, NM 87108
(505) 266-0911
(800) 545-2437 (In-state only)

New Mexico AIDS Services
1223 St. Francis Drive, Suite C
Santa Fe, NM 87501
(505) 984-0911
(800) 545-2437 Hotline (In-state only)

North Carolina

AIDS Community Residence Association (ACRA)
PO Box 61584
Durham, NC 27715
(919) 479-4834

AIDS Control Program
USCDC Dept. of Environmental Health and Natural Resources
Division of Epidemiology, NIV & STDs
PO Box 27687
Raleigh, NC 27611-7687
(919) 733-7301
(800) 342-2437 Nationall AIDS Hotline
(800) 344-7432 National Spanish AIDS Hotline
(800) 243-7889 TDD

The AIDS Service Agency
PO Box 12583
Raleigh, NC 27605
(919) 834-2437

The AIDS Services Project (TASP)
PO Box 3203
Durham, NC 27715-3203
(919) 286-7475

AIDS Task Force of Winston-Salem
PO Box 20983
Winston-Salem, NC 27120
(919) 723-5031
(300) 489-0527

GROW (a Community Service Corporation HIV Services Project)
9441 Highway 117 South
Rocky Point, NC 28457
(919) 675-9222
(800) 732-5432

Metrolina AIDS Project (MAP)
PO Box 32662
Charlotte, NC 28231
(704) 333-1345
(704) 333-2437 Hotline
(800) 289-2437 Hotline (In-state only)

Onslow County AIDS Task Force and Ryan White Program
612 College Street
Jacksonville, NC 28540
(919) 347-2154
(919) 455-3377 Hotline

Triad Health Project
PO Box 5716
Greensboro, NC 27435-0716
(919) 275-1654
(919) 884-4116 Highpoint Office
(800) 868-6785

Western North Carolina AIDS Project
PO Box 2411
Asheville, NC 28802
(800) 346-3731

North Dakota

State Department of Health Division of Disease Control
600 East Boulevard Avenue
Bismarck, ND 58505-0200
(701) 224-2378
(800) 472-2180 (In-state only)
(701) 224-2376 Hotline

Ohio

AIDS Volunteers of Cincinnati
2183 Central Parkway
Cincinnati, OH 45214
(513) 421-2437

Columbus AIDS Task Force
1500 West Third Avenue, Suite 329
Columbus, OH 43212
(614) 488-2437
(800) 332-2437 Hotline (In-state only)
(800) 332-3889 TDD (In-state only)

Health Issues Task Force
2250 Euclid Avenue
Cleaveland, OH 44115
(216) 621-0766

Oklahoma

HIV Resource Center
4154 South Harvard, Suite H-1
Tulsa, OK 74135
(918) 749-4194

Oasis Resources Center
2135 NW 39th
Oklahoma City, OK 73112
(405) 525-AIDS

Oklahoma State Department of Health
HIV/STD Service, Division 0308
1000 NE 10th Street
Oklahoma, OK 73117-1299
(405) 271-4636

Regional AIDS INterfaith Network (RAIN)
4151 South Harvard, Suite H-1
Tulsa, OK 74135
(918) 749-4195

Shanti/Tulsa
PO Box 4318
Tulsa, OK 74159
(918) 749-7898

Oregon

Cascade AIDS Project
408 SW Second Avenue
Portland, OR 97204
(800) 777-2437
(503) 223-5907

Shanti/Oregon
Box 11302
Eugene, OR 97440-3502
(503) 342-5088

Pennsylvania

AIDS Library of Philadelphia
32 North 3rd Street
Philadelphia, PA 19106
(215) 922-5120
(215) 922-7999TDD

CHOICE
1642 Pine Street
Philadelphia, PA 19103
(215) 545-8686
(215) 732-2437 Hotline

Pennsylvania Department of Health
Health and Welfare Building, Room 912
PO Box 90
Harrisburg, PA 17108
(717) 783-0573
(800) 662-6080 Hotline (In-state only)

Philadelphia AIDS Task Force and Resource Library
1216 Walnut Street
Philadelphia, PA 19107
(215) 732-AIDS Hotline

South Central AIDS Assistance Network
2 A Kline Village, Suite A
Harrisburg, PA 17104
(717) 238-2437
(800) 662-6080 Hotline (In-state only)

Puerto Rico

AIDS Central Office
Puerto Rico Department of Health
PO Box 71421
San Juan, PR 00936-8523
(809) 721-2000
(809) 765-1010 Hotline
(800) 981-5721 (PR only)

Foundacion SIDA de Puerto Rico
GPO Box 36-4842
San Juan, PR 00936-4842
(809) 782-9600

Rhode Island

Lifeline
25 Pomona Avenue
Providence, RI 02908
(401) 421-5344

Project AIDS
95 Chestnut Street, 3rd Floor
Providence, RI 02908-4161
(401) 831-5522
(800) 726-3010 Hotline

Stratogen Health
400 Reservoir Avenue
Providence, RI 02907
(401)781-2400
(800) 523-8664 Hotline

South Carolina

Palmetto AIDS Life Support Services of South Carolina (PALSS)
PO Box 12124
Columbia, SC 29211
(803) 779-7257
(800) 723-7257 (In-state only)

South Carolina AIDS Education Network (SCAN)
2768 Decker Boulevard
Columbia, SC 29208
(803) 736-1171

South Carolina Department of Health and Environmental Control, HIV/AIDS Division
PO Box 101106
Columbia, SC 29211
(803) 737-4110
(800) 322-2437 (In-state only)

South Dakota

South Dakota Department of Health AIDS/HIV Project
445 East Capital Avenue
Pierre, SD 57501-3185
(605) 773-3364
(800) 592-1861 Hotline (In-state only)

Tennessee

AIDS Response
PO Box 6069
Knoxville, TN 37914-6069
(615) 523-2437 Hotline

Friends for Life
321 South Bellevue
Memphis, TN 38104
(901) 727-0855

Human Beings Care
PO Box 3339
Jackson, TN 38303
(901) 423-0330
(800)562-3383 Hotline

Tennessee Department of Health AIDS Program
C0221 Cordell Hull Building
Nashville, TN 37247-4947
(615) 741-7500
(800) 525-2437 Hotline (In-state only)

Texas

AIDS Foundation of Houston
3202 Wesleyan Annex
Houston, TX 77027
(713) 623-6796
(713) 524-2437 Hotline

AIDS Helpline for Health Professionals
University of Texas Health Science Center
PO Box 20186
Houston, TX 77225
(713) 794-1760
(800) 548-4659 Hotline

AIDS Services of Austin
PO Box 4874
Austin, TX 78765
(512) 451-2273
(800) 458-2437 Hotline

City of Houston HIV/AIDS Hotline
8000 North Stadium Drive
Houston, TX 77054
(713) 794-9092
(713) 794-9020 Hotline

Dallas AIDS Resource Center
2701 Regan Street
Dallas, TX 75219
(214) 559-2437 Hotline
(214) 521 5124

Informa SIDA
1643 East 2nd Street
Austin, TX 78702
(512) 472-2001 Bilingual line

Texas Deparrtment of Health Texas AIDSLINE
1100 West 49th Street
Austin, TX 78756
(512) 458-7400
(800) 299-2437 Hotline (In-state only)

Valley AIDS Council
2220 Haine Drive, Suite 33
Harlingen, TX 78550
(210) 428-9322
(800) 333-7432 Hotline

Utah

Utah AIDS Foundation
1408 South 1100 E
Salt Lake City, UT 84105
(801)- 487-2323
(801) 487-2100 Hotline
(800) 366-2437 Hotline (in-state only)

Vermont

Vermont Cares
PO Box 5248
Burlington, VT 05402-5243
(802) 863-2437
(800) 649-2437 Hotline (In-state only)

Vermont State Department of Health
The AIDS Program
PO Box 70
Burlington, VT 05402
(802) 863-7245
(800) 882-2437 Hotline (In-state only)

Virginia

Richmond AIDS Information Network
1721 Hanover Avenue
Richmond, VA 23220
(804) 358-2437
(804) 358-8538 Clinic
(804) 358-6434 Hotline

Richmond AIDS Ministry (RAM)
2403 West Main Street
Richmond, VA 23220
(804) 359-4616

Virginia Department of Health STD/AIDS Hotline
PO Box 2448
Richmond, VA 23218
(804) 225-3896
(804) 371-7455 Hotline
(800) 371-7455 Hotline (In-state only)

Virgin Islands

Department of Health
Virgin Islands-St. Thomas HIV Project
St. Tomas Island, VI 00802
(809) 774-3168

Washington

Northwest AIDS Foundation
127 Broadway East, Suite 200
Seattle, WA 98102-5711
(206) 329-6923
(206) 329-6923 Hotline

Shanti/Seattle
PO Box 20698
Seattle, WA 98102
(206) 322-0279

Washington State HIV/AIDS Hotline
MS 47840
Airdustrial Park Building 9
Olympia, WA 98504-0406
(206) 586-3887
(800) 272-2437 Hotline (In-state only)

West Virginia

Huntington AIDS Task Force
824 Fifth Avenue
Huntington, WV 25704
(304) 522-4357
(800) HELP-522

Mountain State AIDS Network
PO Box 1221
235 High Street, Suite 306
Morgantown, WV 26505
(304) 292-9000
(800) 585-4444 Hotline

Ruby Memorial Hospital HIV Clinic
West Virginia University
Morgantown, WV 26505
(304) 293-3306

Wisconsin

AIDS Resource Center of Wisconsin
315 West Court Street
Milwaukee, WI 53212
(414) 273-1991
(414) 273-2437 Hotline
(800) 334-2437 Hotline (In-state only)

Wyoming

Wyoming AIDS Hotline
Hathaway Building, 4th Floor
2300 Capitol Avenue
Cheyenne, WY 82002-0710
(307) 777-5800
(800) 327-3577 Hotline

Wyoming AIDS Project
PO Box 9353
Caspar, WY 82609
(307) 237-7833
(800) 327-3577 Hotline

1993 Revised Classification System for HIV Infection[1] and Expanded AIDS Surveillance Case Definition for Adolescents and Adults[2]			
	Clinical Categories		
CD_4 T-cell Ranges	(A) Asymptomatic, Acute, (primary) HIV or PGL[3]	(B) Symptomatic, Not (A) or (C) Conditions	(C) AIDS-Indicator Conditions
(1) $\geq$ 500/μL	A1	B1	C1
(2) 200-499/μL	A2	B2	C2
(3) < 200/μL	A3	B3	C3

1 Criteria for HIV infection for persons $\geq$ 13 years: a) repeatedly reactive screening to test for HIV antibody (e.g., enzyme immunoassay) with specific antibody identified by the use of supplemental tests (e.g., Western blot, immunofluorescence assay); b) direct identification of virus in host tissues by virus isolation; c) HIV antigen detection; or d) a positive result on any other highly specific licensed test for HIV.

2 The shaded cells illustrate the expanded AIDS surveillance case definition. Persons with AIDS-indicator condition (Category C) as well as those with CD_4 T-cell Ranges < 200/μL (Categories A3 or B3) are reportable as AIDS cases in the United States and Territories , effective January 1, 1993.

3 PGL is Persistent Generalized Lymphadenopathy.

Clinical Conditions Included in the 1993 Revised AIDS Surveillance Case Definition:

- *Candidiasis of bronchi, trachea or lungs;*
- *Candidiasis, esophageal;*
- *Cervical cancer, invasive;*
- *Coccidioidomycosis, disseminated or extrapulmonary;*
- *Cryptococcosis, extrapulmonary;*
- *Cryptosporidiosis, chronic intestinal, > 1 month duration;*
- *Cytomegalovirus disease, other than liver, spleen or nodes;*
- *Cytomegalovirus retinitis, with loss of vision;*
- *Encephalopathy, HIV-related;*
- *Herpes simplex: chronic ulcer(s), > 1 month duration or bronchitis, pneumonitis or esophagitis;*
- *Histoplasmosis, disseminated or extrapulmonary;*
- *Isoporiasis, chronic intestinal, > 1 month duration;*
- *Kaposi's sarcoma;*
- *Lymphoma, Burkitt's, or equivalent term;*
- *Lymphoma, immunoblastic, or equivalent term;*
- *Lymphoma, primary in brain;*
- *Mycobacterium avium complex or M. kansasii, disseminated or extrapulmonary;*
- *Mycobacterium tuberculosis, any site, pulmonary or extrapulmonary;*
- *Pneumonia, recurrent;*
- *Progressive multifocal leukoencephalopathy;*
- *Salmonella* septicemia, recurrent;
- Toxoplasmosis of brain;
- Wasting syndrome due to HIV.

(Adapted from the MMWR, December 18, 1992 (Vol. 41, No. RR-17).